Music Therapy With Premature Infants: Research and Developmental Interventions

Music Therapy
With Premature Infants:
Research and Developmental Interventions

Jayne M. Standley, Ph.D., MT-BC
The Florida State University

The American Music Therapy Association, Inc.

The American Music Therapy Association is a non-profit association dedicated to increasing access to quality music therapy services for individuals with disabilities or illnesses or for those who are interested in personal growth and wellness. AMTA provides extensive educational and research information about the music therapy profession. Referrals for qualified music therapists are also provided to consumers and parents. AMTA holds an annual conference every autumn and its eight regions hold conferences every spring.

For up-to-date information, please access the AMTA website at www.musictherapy.org

ISBN: 1-884914-09-8

The American Music Therapy Association, Inc.
8455 Colesville Road, Suite 1000
Silver Spring, MD 20910

Phone: (301) 589-3300
Fax: (301) 589-5175
Email: info@musictherapy.org
Website: www.musictherapy.org

Photos graciously provided by — Nikki Elliott.
Cover design — Ann Karns Aiken.
Technical assistance — Wordsetters, Inc.
Layout design and formatting — Angie K Elkins.

Printed in The United States of America

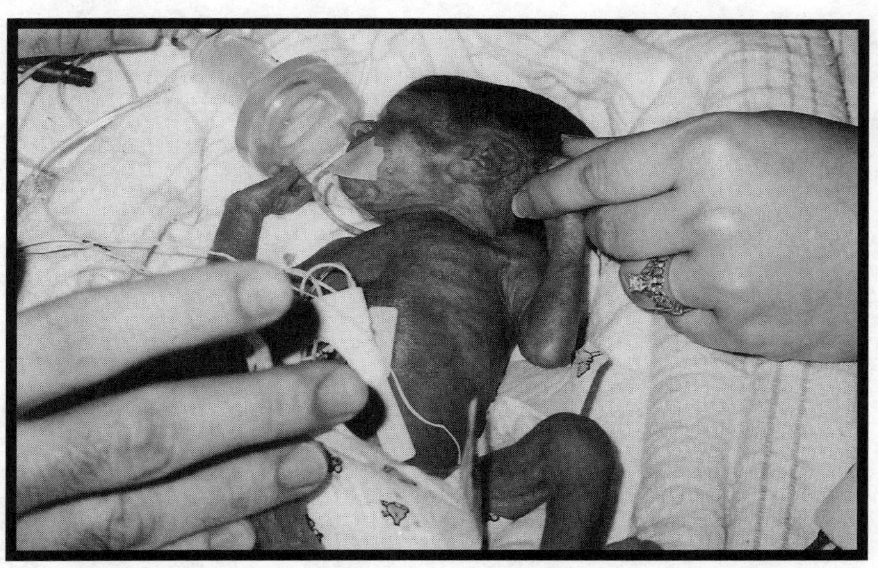

This book is dedicated to Libby, born at 26-27 weeks gestation, 1 pound, 11 ounces (771 grams) and to her music therapist Mom, Nikki Elliott.

Contents

List of Tables

List of Figures

Acknowledgments

Many persons contributed to the publication of this volume. I am deeply indebted to the medical staff of Tallahassee Memorial Hospital, the site where the bulk of research with music therapy and premature infants was conducted. All of the personnel in the Newborn Intensive Care Unit gave willingly of their expertise and provided invaluable assistance to research projects. I am especially grateful to Sherry Wisham, RNC, Head Nurse of the NBICU, whose vision for improved infant care afforded opportunity for innovative clinical trials. And to the many parents who allowed their precious infants to participate in this research, I am profoundly appreciative.

I am indebted to the Center for Music Research in the School of Music and to Florida State University (FSU) for support of my research. My esteemed colleague, Dr. Clifford Madsen, guided my thinking when I first delved into the area of infant research in 1986. Eitaro Kawaguchi of the Center for Music Research engineered the original PAL, the pacifier-activated-lullaby mechanism. Ross Henderson of the FSU Psychology Department consulted in its design. John Frasier, Director of Technology Transfer, obtained a patent for the device. Jack Sams, Senior Licensing Manager, provided licensing liaison and assisted in acquiring development funds.

Susan Mazer and Dallas Smith of Healing Healthcare Systems, Inc. are currently developing the PAL for marketing by Ohmeda

Medical, Inc. They provided prototypes for ongoing research and recorded the special musical arrangements we used. William R. Mandel, engineer of the prototypes, kept us supplied with transmitters and was our troubleshooter for all problems. Sassy Products provided pacifiers for the original PAL device and Children's Medical Venture, Inc. provided pacifiers for the prototypes. I thank them all for their interest and commitment to the PAL and for the excellent working relationships we have enjoyed.

I wish to thank my friend and colleague, Dr. Jane Cassidy of Louisiana State University, whose innovative research on the hearing ability of premature infants has provided critical information for the provision of auditory stimuli for therapeutic benefit. She is always available to support, discuss, and encourage new ideas for research.

I am most grateful to Jennifer Whipple, MT-BC, the first music therapist at TMH who masterfully initiated clinical MT programs, internships, student practica, arts in medicine volunteer opportunities, and research projects in a very short interval of time. Her coordination of the NICU MT program was helpful in recent years in collection of data. She also gave freely of her expertise for editorial review of the manuscript during its preparation and provided the Glossary of Medical Terms for this volume.

I wish also to thank Darcy Walworth, MT-BC, the second music therapist at TMH, for her support and assistance in the acquisition of NICU research subjects, for ongoing coordination of the NICU MT programs, and for continued development of the TMH MT program into unique and creative clinical areas. To all of the Florida State University music therapy students who have volunteered over the last 5 years in the daily NICU Infant Stimulation program, my grateful appreciation.

Finally, to Nikki Elliott, music therapist and mom, who shared the wonderful pictures of the development of her premature infant daughter, Libby, I am most appreciative.

Preface

This book is the synthesis of over 20 years of music therapy research with premature infants and infant learning. It is intended to collect in one volume the current state of research findings in NICU music therapy and to interpret those findings for the responsible application of clinical programs to enhance the development of the fragile, pre-term infant. The music use advocated in these pages is clearly documented by experimental investigation.

It is exciting to realize that the body of research reported here shows music therapy to provide many physiological, behavioral, and developmental benefits for premature infants while revealing a distinct absence of adverse side effects when care is taken for control of volume, duration, and type of music stimuli. In the investigation of new areas of medical treatment, such findings are rare. This text is intended for the use of qualified music therapists, neonatal specialists, and/or parents of premature infants. It is hoped that it will aid and benefit the children for whom they care.

The treatment of premature infants has made great strides in the last 10 years. Much is known about the detrimental effects of lack of appropriate environmental and nurturing stimulation during medical treatment. Much is still to be learned about the safest, most effective ways to involve NICU infants in human interaction. Music therapy has long been one of the key components of an effective curriculum for infant stimulation and for teaching children with developmental disabilities. It is encouraging that the medical community is beginning to embrace music therapy as an important contribution to safe and effective infant stimulation at the onset of life, even when that life begins without full gestational development.

This text marks the emergence of the development of NICU music therapy programs and, while strongly based in research, it is only a small beginning. As the field grows, it is obvious that ongoing effort is needed to provide greater diversity and databases with much larger sample sizes. It is also obvious that the need for long-term, follow-up research is critical. It is hoped that this text will precipitate interest in continued investigation and development in music therapy with premature infants.

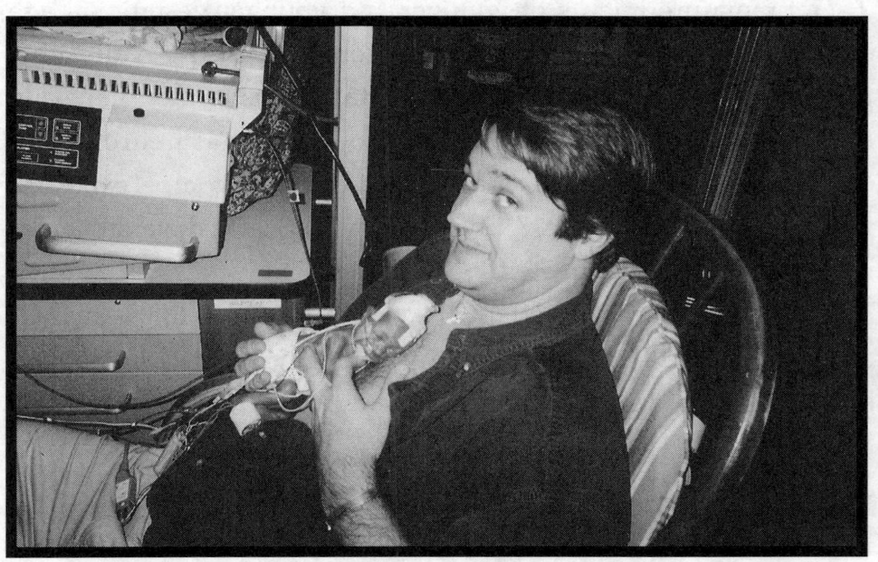

During the Cautious Stimulation Phase of development, Mom and Dad can begin skin-to-skin kangaroo care that helps Libby thrive and promotes bonding. Other touch or movement is not yet recommended.

1 | Third Trimester Fetal Development

As health care and medical technology improve, seriously premature infants of younger and younger gestational age survive an early birth. Many such survivors complete the entire third trimester of development in the neonatal intensive care unit. This outside-the-womb maturation interrupts normal neurological development and the fragile infant's medical needs compel exposure to trauma, pain and stress. A potential for long-term developmental complications is thus created.

Unlike the premature infant, the term baby enters life as an avid and experienced learner equipped with beginning discriminations and memory of language, emotional response, and awareness of cause/effect relationships. This learning began in the womb and continues rapidly from birth.

To prevent lifelong developmental complications, the premature infant's learning process must begin at birth and continue during his/her stay in the Neonatal Intensive Care Unit (NICU). Music shows promise for soothing and nurturing premature infants, reducing stress, stabilizing physiological functions and behavior states, and promoting language exposure, thus enhancing maturation during this critical final stage of fetal development under medical treatment. The purpose of this book is to summarize current research on pre/perinatal neurological growth, infant learning, and music therapy in the NICU and to describe research-based clinical applications for music therapy developmental intervention with premature infants during the first year of life.

Normal Neurological Development in the Third Trimester

Magnetic resonance imaging (MRI) allows observation and analysis of the functioning human brain and reveals astonishing new information about its early development (Roush, 1997). Scientists feel that they have learned more in the last 10 years about neurological development than was previously known throughout history. For instance, it has recently been discovered that during fetal development the Right side of the brain grows faster and will usually favor the more primitive human attributes. Further along in gestation, the Left side of the brain starts growing and will eventually perform those human behaviors acquired later in evolution, such as language (Chiron et al., 1997; Kotulak, 1993). In the third trimester, the human fetus is adding 250,000 neurons/minute in the developing brain. During this period 100 billion neurons will form, all a human will get throughout a lifetime. During fetal development and at birth, these neural cells compete with each other connecting across tiny spaces called synapses to link up with a specific neurological function (Fischer & Rose, 1994). In order to become permanent, these connections must be used regularly. By a normal term birth, half of these cells will already have become dysfunctional due to failure to link to a purpose. The newborn's brain is about 1/3 the size of an adult's but will triple in size by age 2 years.

The central nervous system is still quite immature at birth and continues rapid, critical development in the first year of life. Learning and intelligence derive from each individual's unique combination of endowed genetics and environmental opportunity to acquire information. The newborn is, therefore, self-constructing with neonatal and post birth experiences creating the particular connections for each individual. The brain requires stimulation (touch, sound, movement, and hearing) to develop and will go through four periods of major structural change: during fetal development, after birth, from ages 4-10, and during the remainder of life. From birth to age 3 most of the neurological "wiring" takes place. Cells compete for function and, finding none, will die off, re-commit to a new purpose, or simply fail to align in useful, functional patterns (Kotulak, 1993). The need for rapid development of brain function makes the predicament of premature infants particularly vulnerable with early intervention being imperative to assist their developmental progression.

Neurons have restricted windows of developmental opportunity for some functions mandating that stimulation must occur at the correct times or effective skills will never emerge. Vision function is critical from birth to 6 months while speech and language skills must be presented prior to 3 years of age. From ages 4-10 years the brain becomes very dense from the great many connections that have been formed. At around age 11, the brain begins eliminating unused wiring to increase the power and efficiency of its circuitry.

As the infant matures, neurological development will progress cephalocaudally (from the head down) and proximodistally (from the center of the body out to the periphery). The infant will move from gross to fine motor coordination and will achieve head control, trunk control, and arm and grasping control prior to walking. Cognition will progress from awareness of stimuli, to sustained attention across time called tracking, to discrimination among stimuli and, finally, to more and more complex associations and conceptualizations within the environment. The infant will learn skills which activate and utilize multiple areas of the brain such as those in language and those in music which simultaneously combine sensory perception, cognition, and motor ability.

Gender Differences in Development

It is now theorized that all fetal brains begin with female characteristics. If the infant is to be a male, an infusion of testosterone changes the brain, establishing male characteristics at the same time in prenatal development when the two parts of the brain have the greatest difference in growth. These discoveries have provided rationale for theories of why more males than females exhibit Left side neurological dysfunction such as stuttering, dyslexia, and language disorders (Kotulak, 1993). At term birth, females are more developed with regard to hearing (Cassidy & Ditty, 2001), have better tactile and oral sensitivity, and are more responsive to smiling, sweet tastes, talking, eye-to-eye contact and to the pacifier. Cerebral blood flow in girls is significantly lower than in males. Male infants demonstrate more startles, more muscle activity, and more physical strength.

With regard to auditory capability at birth, male infants actually have shorter cochlea, fewer hair cells and less response to aural stimuli. Female infants hear high frequencies better than males which is particularly advantageous when listening to music with its wide range of frequencies (Cassidy & Ditty, 2001).

Hearing Development

The potential for music benefit to premature infants evolved when it was determined that auditory stimuli are perceived and discriminated by the fetus early in development (Cheour-Luhtanen et al., 1996). It has been documented that as early as 18 weeks gestational age, loud sounds cause the fetal heart rate to increase and at 25 weeks the major structures of the ear are essentially in place. At 25-27 gestation weeks most fetuses begin to respond inconsistently to sound by moving or kicking. But this response quickly fatigues. Researchers are convinced that hearing is functioning by 29 gestation weeks when the normally developing fetus consistently responds to auditory stimuli. At this time the auditory thresholds are quite high and begin to decrease from the 26th to 35th weeks of gestation age. At 35 weeks auditory thresholds are close to adult levels.

During the third trimester, auditory ranges are restricted (500-1000 Hz) compared to those for term infants (approximately 500-4000 Hz) and adults (30-20,000 Hz) (Roeser, 1996). It is theorized that this lower range concentrates the fetus's ability in the area of speech frequencies (500-3000 Hz) for language development (Glass, 1994).

It is now known that the 30-35 gestation week fetus is hearing maternal and nearby environmental sounds and beginning to respond. It has also been demonstrated that this auditory input while in the womb is assimilated and learned. The fetus begins to discriminate among speech sounds, particularly with regard to pitch and rhythm (Lecanuet, Granier-Deferre, & Busnel, 1995). At birth, the term infant demonstrates that he/she recognizes the mother's voice, prefers women's voices over men's voices, recognizes stories and melodies heard during the final trimester of development, and recognizes his/her native language (DeCasper & Fifer, 1980; DeCasper & Spence, 1986; Kolata, 1984, Moon, Cooper, & Fifer, 1993, Polverini-Rey, 1992).

Some researchers have investigated responses to intrauterine music exposure. Shetler (1989) identified four infants who were regularly and systematically exposed to music while in the womb. All were observed postnatally between the ages of 21-47 months and were described at that point as demonstrating singing ability and interest in music. Such a small sample size would not allow generalization to the assumption that all infants hearing music in the womb would be interested in music later, though this is an intriguing area for further research and may have implication for positive benefits of early or premature music exposure.

Woodward and colleagues presented a specific music selection prenatally and then tested its reinforcement potential against other musical selections after the birth of the infant (Woodward et al, 1992). They demonstrated that the presented music was more reinforcing to the newborn, thereby indicating memory and recognition. In a similar vein, Polverini-Rey (1992) demonstrated that intrauterine lullaby exposure increased the calming response to that lullaby after birth.

As yet, little research exists to document the prenatal development of specific music discriminations for pitch, rhythm, and/or harmony, though existing literature has demonstrated that these abilities are evident within a few months of life (Michel, 1973; Moog, 1976; Ries, 1982; Summers, 1984; Tims, 1978; Wendrich, 1981).

The normal, full-term infant's developmental ability to respond to auditory stimuli has been extensively studied. At birth, it has been documented as a consistent head turn response, which due to neurological immaturity occurs 8-11 seconds following the onset of the stimulus (Muir, 1985). The infant's heart rate also responds to sound. Heart rate deceleration indicates orienting to, or focusing on, an auditory stimulus while infant attention during heart rate acceleration indicates a defensive response, as to stimuli which are aversive, startling, or too loud (Karmel, Gardner, & Magnano, 1991). It should also be noted that responses to auditory stimuli are state dependent (Goff, 1985). A sleeping infant will respond less than will an awake or alert infant. It is evident that continued auditory exposure from birth contributes to the further development, complexity, and specification of auditory abilities (Lecanuet et al., 1995).

It is still unclear what appropriate auditory guidelines would be for premature infants at various stages of development and for various types of sound. It is known that premature infants have elevated hearing thresholds until reaching full term development. However, sound after birth is transmitted via air, not buffered by conduction through amniotic fluid. Therefore, the same sounds outside are received with greater intensity than inside the womb.

Most NICU environments, unfortunately, have constant ambient noise at high dB levels 24 hours per day. Ambient noise masks speech input to the infant and causes stress responses (American Academy of Pediatrics, 1997). Prolonged exposure to high aberrant noise levels may even contribute to impaired language development (Glass, 1994). Other sounds, like music and the human voice, are acoustically different from noise and are perceived as less stressful, though fatiguing if their duration or complexity are too great. Auditory stimuli should be carefully controlled and monitored as guidelines continue to develop from the research literature.

Implications of Premature Infant Development in the NICU

In the United States, the medical diagnosis of low birth weight (LBW) includes those infants born prematurely, prior to 37 weeks gestational age, and those born small for gestational age, below 5 pounds, 8 ounces (2500 grams). The annual incidence of LBW children as of 2000 was 7.6% of the 4.1 million live births, over 307,000 infants per year and, for preterm infants, was 11.6%, over 467,000 births per year. (Martin, Hamilton, Ventura, Menacker, & Park, 2002). Prematurity and low birth weight are the second leading cause of infant mortality. The closer the gestational age at delivery to full-term (38-40 weeks), the greater the probability of survival. With contemporary medical intervention, very premature infants born as early as 24 weeks gestation have a 56% probability of surviving in the U.S. while those born at 32.5 weeks have over 95% survival rate (Centers for Disease Control [CDC], 1999).

The majority of LBW infants (50-60%) will have serious educational difficulties and require special education resources throughout their years in the public school system (Hack, Klein, & Taylor, 1995). Developmental problems will be greatest for infants with a birth weight less than 1500 grams or born prior to 32 weeks gestation. Very premature infants have a high probability of long-term, impaired neurological development (Horbar & Lucey, 1995). Recent research has demonstrated that preterm infants will develop smaller brain volume and more limited cognitive abilities than term infants (Peterson et al., 2000). They also will have decreased growth attainment throughout the developing years.

Though learning impairments are life-long, medical costs far outweigh the educational costs related to this problem in the U.S. Care for LBW infants comprises 10% of all health care costs for children in this country (CDC, 1999). Premature infants stay in highly specialized neonatal intensive or intermediate care units (NICU) until they achieve a body weight of approximately 4 to 4.5 pounds which usually coincides with their original due date. The cost/child for initial hospitalization averages $33,000 compared with that for term infants of $1,900. Low birth weight children are twice as likely to be hospitalized during early childhood and, when hospitalized, will stay there longer (Lewit, Baker, Corman, & Shiono, 1995). Their physiological problems include respiratory immaturity and organ immaturity, especially of the heart, lungs, kidneys, and bowels. Other common medical problems include asthma, upper and lower respiratory infections, and ear infections.

The proliferation and sophistication of NICUs have increased greatly in the last 10 years and it is estimated that there are now more than 700 throughout the United States (Horbar & Lucey, 1995).

Research has shown that NICU development has lowered premature infant fatalities dramatically. Individual hospital factors that contribute to premature infant survival include use of APGAR scores, large number of delivery services, greater than average number of Cesarean sections, and status as a Level III hospital. As special NICU procedures have developed, disagreement still exists as to when to intervene, when to resuscitate, and what treatment procedures to provide.

Some learning problems are caused by the treatment procedures necessary for survival and subsequent negative side effects. High levels of oxygen cause retrolental fibroplasia, a permanent visual impairment. Some of the drugs given to the infant are ototoxic, causing permanent hearing loss. Additionally, the ambient sound levels in the incubator and NICU environment are aversive and stressful sometimes measuring as high as 75-80 dB (Scale A). Premature infants may be subjected to these sounds for 24 hours/day for as long as several months. Many premature infants will later develop hyperactivity, specific learning disabilities or attention deficit disorders. It is theorized that persistently high stress levels during medical treatment contribute to these neurological impairments (Creasey, Jarvis, Myers, Markowitz, & Kerkering, 1991). Unfortunately, stress and trauma elevate levels of the hormone cortisol, which floods the brain. This cortisol excess contributes to a 20-30% reduced growth in tissue in some regions of the brain.

Medical Care of the Premature Infant

Premature infants require highly specialized care in settings with trained personnel and equipment. Premature infants born in areas with only Level I hospitals (basic care) will be transported immediately to a Level II (specialty care) NICU. Those with unusual and severe medical complications will be sent to a Level III (subspecialty) facility. Such transport is lifesaving, but may interfere with parental visitation, bonding, and participation in developmental therapies. Premature infants will remain in the NICU until their approximate due date, so the most severely premature (23-24 weeks) will be hospitalized for three months or longer.

Immediately upon birth the infant will be placed in the high risk nursing area for initial assessments and observation. Progress will be monitored according to gestational age and individual medical problems. When the infant's need for mechanical respiration support and serious medical problems are resolved, he/she will be promoted to intermediate care status. Infants in intermediate care are informally known as "growers and feeders" meaning they are progressing nicely and are remaining under specialized care until maturation and growth reach minimal levels for discharge. The earliest at which discharge usually occurs is around 34 weeks and is dependent upon whether the infant is maintaining body temperature, nipple feeding, and consistently gaining weight. Also, parents must be trained and feel comfortable in caring for the special needs of the child.

Most medical personnel feel that the earliest discharge possible is best for the infant even though he/she may go home with daily electronic and home monitoring by trained professionals. When all supports and resources are present, infants usually thrive better in the more benign home environment than in the hospital NICU environment. It is not unusual for the infant to have to occasionally return to the hospital for care or solution of specific problems that develop across time. This is still considered to be more developmentally beneficial and is less costly than remaining in the hospital for longer periods at the beginning of life.

Medical Assessments

During the initial period in neonatal intensive care, the survival of the seriously premature infant is of paramount concern.

Assessments of developmental and medical status are made and a medical treatment plan formulated. The infant is assessed at birth on the APGAR Scale and then 24 hours later on a determination of maturation and gestation age (GA) such as the Dubowitz Scale or the New Ballard Score (see Appendix). The infant is also medically examined for a variety of complications of prematurity.

APGAR. APGAR is an acronym for five categories of infant behavior and physiology assessed at birth to ascertain the need for immediate life-sustaining assistance (Garcia-Prats & Hornfischer, 2000). The APGAR score ranges from 0-10 points and is assessed at 1 minute after birth for tolerance to the birth process and at 5 minutes after birth to assess adaptation to the environment. A third assessment is done at 10 minutes if deemed necessary. The APGAR scores are usually reported sequentially, as in APGARs of 7 and 9. Zero to 2 points are awarded in each of 5 categories then totaled for the score as shown in Table 1. A normal APGAR is 8-10 points with less than 8 points indicating that the infant needed some assistance adapting to the post-birth environment. A score of 10 is very unusual since almost all newborns lose 1 point for blue hands and feet. An APGAR score of less than 4 usually indicates that the infant needed some resuscitation to survive. APGAR scores at birth correlate highly with ongoing developmental outcomes.

Table 1. APGAR Assessment

Categories	0 points	1 point	2 points
Appearance	Pale blue	Pink body with blue extremities	Entire body is pink (unusual)
Pulse	No heart beat	<100 bpm	>100 bpm
Grimace	None	Grimacing	Vigorous cry
Activity/Tone	Flaccid muscle tone	Some flexion of extremities	Active motion
Respiration	No respiration effort	Slow, irregular respiration	Crying with normal respiration

Growth Factors. The average birth weight for a full-term infant is between 7 and 8 pounds. The earliest gestational age at birth at which survival is likely (50%) is around 24 weeks and babies born at this time usually weigh around 1 pound. Weight of premature infants is often reported in grams (g) or kilograms (k=1000g). A conversion table is used to translate grams to pounds and ounces (see Appendix). One ounce is equal to approximately 28g and 1 pound is about 454g. Infants lose weight during the first few days after birth and then slowly start to gain. Those who are thriving after 34 weeks gestation usually gain around 1 ounce/day. Average weight for discharge is usually close to 4.5 pounds.

Male and female infants differ widely in normative data for growth factors. Males weigh more at birth than females, but are neurologically more immature. Females tend to mature and thrive faster than males. Therefore, all analyses of typical growth and development are differentiated by gender. The infant's weight and length are regularly plotted on charts with normal growth curve parameters by age and gender. Thus, it is immediately apparent if the infant's growth data deviate from these norms. (See Appendix for growth charts.)

The length of the infant will be measured at birth and periodically throughout the NICU stay to assess overall growth and the relationship between weight and length. The head circumference will be measured at birth and weekly thereafter to ascertain whether fluid accumulation from intraventricular bleeds or hydrocephalus is developing. Physical examination will assess the infant's muscle tone, symmetry of posture, and limb position.

Monitors. Special equipment will be used to monitor the infant's physiological status 24 hours/day. Most common are the cardiorespiratory or heart monitor, the pulse oximeter, and temperature probe. These are noninvasive and will be attached by adhesive electrodes to the infant's skin on the chest and extremities. The heart monitor measures heart and immediate respiration rate and patterns across time. It sounds an alarm if the infant's heart stops beating, beats very irregularly, or the infant stops breathing.

The pulse oximeter measures blood oxygen saturation, the amount of oxygen in the red blood cells, and sounds an alarm when oxygen saturation falls below 87% or consistently stays above 95%. This allows the respiratory therapist to carefully adjust oxygen levels for the minimal amount necessary.

A temperature sensor is placed on an extremity and connected to the incubator warmer to assure the infant's body temperature remains stable and warm enough. He/she must mature enough to maintain body temperature without mechanical assistance. This usually occurs between 30 and 32 weeks GA and at least several days after birth.

Intravenous Lines. An intravenous (IV) line will be inserted into the infant to deliver life sustaining fluids (total parenteral nutrition and lipids) and medications. These may be superficial, short-term insertions just under the skin which last from 2-4 days or may be a central line inserted directly into a large vein in the scalp, leg, or arm which is designed to last for several weeks (Garcia-Prats & Hornfischer, 2000). Sometimes an umbilical catheter is inserted into the umbilical artery for drawing blood or giving transfusions. All IV insertions are potential sites for development of infection and are carefully monitored by medical staff.

Arterial Blood Gas Tests. If the baby is on assisted respiration blood gas tests are essential for maintaining a balance between oxygen and carbon dioxide levels in the blood and also pH levels, the balance of acid/base factors (Garcia-Prats & Hornfischer, 2000). Arterial blood gas tests are made several times daily during assisted ventilation. Adjustments to oxygen levels and respiratory assistance will be made by the Respiratory Therapist according to these tests.

Sensory Evaluations. Eye exams will be given at several points during treatment to assess development of any visual problems (retinoptahy of prematurity, nystagmus, cataracts, etc.). Correction will probably be done immediately since the window for neurological development of effective vision is very short. Sometimes, premature infants leave the NICU already wearing corrective lenses.

A screening for hearing ability will be given just prior to discharge. Some drugs critical to the infant's survival are ototoxic and place the infant at high risk for hearing loss. The screening identifies those infants who require further assessment and observation to assure effective language development.

Nutritional Issues. The infant will probably be fed the first few days or weeks intravenously. Typically a mixture of sugar, vitamins, minerals and proteins called total parenteral nutrition (TPN), and lipids, free fatty acids, are given initially (Garcia-Prats & Hornfischer, 2000). When the infant's intestines are mature enough to process food, he/she will be fed formula or breast milk by naso-gastric tube until about 34 weeks gestatation. At this age, the ability for a coordinated suck-swallow-breathe response develops. Now the infant is ready for nippling, directly feeding from the breast or bottle.

When the infant is mature enough to process food, breast milk is preferred to formula due to its multiple and dramatic benefits for the premature infant. The breast milk of mothers delivering prematurely contains more fat and nutrition than normal (Garcia-Prats & Hornfischer, 2000). All breast milk contains antibodies to protect the infant from disease, is more easily digested than formula, and has reduced probability for development of allergies.

Breast milk can be expressed by the mother via pumping and delivered to the hospital. It is then stored for subsequent feeding. As the mother continues to pump throughout her infant's NICU stay, she maintains the ability to begin breastfeeding when the infant achieves 34 weeks GA. Most pediatricians recommend providing breast milk to infants for at least the first year of life to maximize the multiple benefits.

Behavior States. At term, infant behavior and consciousness are clearly differentiated into six recognizable levels or states moving from sound sleep to active alertness. The deepest sleep is referred to as quiet sleep. The infant's eyelids are closed and unmoving while its face is relaxed. A less restful sleep is referred to as active sleep which usually occurs in 30-minute cycles. Infants have closed eyes, but their eyelids occasionally flutter. They also frequently make chewing motions or move their face. Drowsiness is the third state and occurs between going to sleep and waking up. The infant is quiet with expressions of smiling or frowning and a dull, glazed look in the eyes. There are two alert states called quiet alert and active alert. Quiet alert is a good time for play and can last up to 30 minutes or longer. The infant's eyes are wide open and he/she will pay close attention to stimuli in the environment. Active alert state is characterized by rapid, frequent movement and is more hyperactive than quiet alert. The baby is usually trying to control large muscle groups for adaptive purposes. The final state is crying which occurs during hunger or discomfort. Shortly after birth, a term infant can make smooth transitions between behavioral states. For instance, crying ceases quickly when the infant is presented with food. Due to neurological immaturity, premature infants can get "stuck" in a behavioral state and have difficulty making a transition on their own. Sometimes assistance must be given by physically moving the infant's body into a more relaxed position.

Ultrasound/Sonagrams/X-Rays. Sonagram or ultrasound tests are a noninvasive way to assess internal issues and the infant's organs. Brain scans assess intraventricular hemorrhage (IVH) or abnormal brain anatomy. Heart ultrasounds identify heart murmurs and abnormal heart or blood vessel anatomy, such as patent ductus arteriosus (PDA). X-rays are used to assess bone formation and air-filled structures such as the lungs and intestines.

Medical Complications of Premature Birth

The very premature infant's need for survival outside the womb prior to adequate development for such survival creates multiple medical complications. Many of these are life threatening and require immediate medical intervention.

Respiratory distress syndrome (RDS) also known as hyaline membrane disease (HMD) is the most common disorder of neonates in the first hours of life (Garcia-Prats & Hornfischer, 2000). It is most frequent in premature infants who weigh less than 1500g at birth (Klaus & Fanaroff, 1993). Placing the infant on a ventilator or respirator and administering a dose of surfactant is the usual treatment. Because of the immaturity of their lungs, some of these infants will also develop a chronic lung condition, bronchopulmonary dysplasia (BPD). Duration of time on the ventilator and probability of BPD are highly correlated. Bronchopulmonary dysplasia is a condition of pressure-induced damage to the lungs and results in long-term breathing difficulties which may require supplemental oxygen upon discharge. Additionally, the tendency for accumulation of fluid in the lungs may result in respiratory infections such as respiratory syncytial virus (RSV) which can be life threatening.

Oxygen toxicity to the blood vessels of the retina of the eye can result in retinopathy of prematurity (ROP) and permanent visual impairment (Spitzer, 1996). The retinal blood vessels are not permanently formed until 40-44 weeks of gestation and are very susceptible to excessive levels of oxygen. With very premature infants, it is a delicate balance to supply enough oxygen to sustain life without damaging the developing visual ability.

Infections (early or late onset) may develop from pre-existing conditions at birth, exposure during extended labor, or from factors associated with the NICU treatment such as IV sites and environmental exposure. Symptoms include intolerance for feedings, lethargy, poor temperature regulation, low blood pressure, apnea, etc.

Apnea occurs when the infant fails to breathe within 15 to 30 seconds and the heart rate drops. The baby's skin changes in color from pink to dusky gray or blue. This is caused by immaturity of the central nervous system and is treated by tapping the infant or the incubator for arousal and to elicit breathing. If this is insufficient, oxygen will be administered, and, if necessary, more extreme resuscitation measures will be employed.

Jaundice is relatively common among premature infants due to immaturity of the liver. It results from excess bilirubin in the body and is treated with a blue fluorescent light. The infant will be placed under the "bili-light" wearing only a diaper and his/her eyes will be protected with a mask. Very severe cases of jaundice may require blood transfusions to prevent damage to the infant's developing brain (Garcia-Prats & Hornfischer, 2000).

Intraventricular hemorrhage, bleeding in the brain, is seen in approximately 40% of infants born at less than 1500g (Watt, 1994). These hemorrhages are graded in four levels with Grade IV having the worst prognosis. Grade I and II bleeds may resolve themselves with little treatment while Grade III and IV bleeds often lead to permanent neurological damage. Excessive bleeding creates blockages and pressure. Sometimes hydrocephalus results and requires installation of a shunt to drain accumulating fluids. In the long term, the majority of infants with hemorrhages at Grades III and IV will have serious neurological deficits, most usually cerebral palsy.

Patent ductus arteriosus (PDA) is an immature condition of the blood vessel connecting the aorta and pulmonary artery that does not allow it to close as it should (Garcia-Prats & Hornfischer, 2000). In the fetus, this vessel is open so that blood bypasses the lungs while they are filled with amniotic fluid. After full-term births, the vessel spontaneously closes within 1-2 days to allow for proper oxygenation of the lungs. Symptoms of PDA include difficulty breathing, irregular vital signs, and a noticeable heart murmur detected externally with a stethoscope.

Necrotizing enterocolitis (NEC) develops after the infant begins feedings. It is an inflammation of the intestinal tract and is characterized by abdominal distention, feeding intolerance, vomiting, bloody stools, and other symptoms of infection (Garcia-Prats & Hornfischer, 2000). If it is serious, necrosis (death) of the tissue of the bowels may occur. For this reason, the infant may be given a colostomy to bypass the immature bowels. The bowels will be reconnected at a later date when the infant is more mature and able to process food.

Frequent regurgitation in the infant is called gastroesophageal reflux (GER) and is a problem of the sphincter valve connecting the stomach to the esophogus (Tracy & Maroney, 1999). This regurgitation is a problem when it reduces the infant's nutritional intake and when the regurgitated stomach acid causes pain. GER is usually resolved with age and maturity of the sphincter valve. Prior to this, it can be alleviated by raising the infant's head after feeding, slowing the rate of feeding, or by administering medications for sphincter tone.

Pain is experienced by premature infants but their response to it may vary from that of the term infant. Without the ability to make a vigorous sound, they may not cry at all or the vocal response may show little acoustic change from discomfort to severe pain (Johnston et al., 1999). They will, however, show changes in body movement, breathing rate, and hormone levels.

Extremely premature infants are often born with neurologic disease or degree of neurologic immaturity that is associated with cerebral atrophy (Maalouf et al., 1999). They frequently develop periventricular leukomalacia (PVL), a morbid softening of the tissue around the ventricles of the brain. Magnetic resonance imaging has revealed reduced brain volume by attainment of term gestation age in these infants (Inder et al., 1999). The prognosis for their neurological outcome is extremely poor.

Developmental Timeline by Gestational Age

Adequate NICU care requires consideration of each individual's gestational age (GA). Personnel assiduously observe symptoms and characteristics of each infant to determine if their development in the NICU is consistent with their estimated gestational age and to ascertain their readiness for particular medical procedures or developmental interventions. Thus, awareness of developmental milestones and timelines for the last trimester is essential.

A full-term pregnancy is 38-42 gestational weeks with due date manually calculated by adding 7 days to the first day of the last menstrual period and counting back 3 months (Garcia-Prats & Hornfischer, 2000). This gives the expected date in the following year for the birth. Currently, ultrasound assessment early in the pregnancy when the fetus is growing most rapidly is a more accurate assessment of gestational age and due date.

Developmental Chart for Severely Premature Infants

Gestational Age in Weeks:	23 24 25 26 27 28 29 30 31 32 33 34 35 36 37 38 39 40 41 42
Birth Status:	Preterm-- Full term---------- Post-term
Vision	Eyes re-open--------------------; Visual fixation & tracking @ 10-12"; Brief eye contact
Hearing	Responds to sound; Cartilage develops in pinna; Turns head to sound after 8-11 seconds
Response to Pain	Responds to pain (somewhat slower); Pathways finish myelinating; Full response to pain
Nutrition & Feeding	IV feeding; Gavage feeding; Suck/swallow/breathe coordinated response; Nippling; Rooting/gagging responses
Social Responses	"In turning"/survival level------------------------; Avoids eye contact; "Coming out"; Tests eye contact intermittently; Reciprocity; Smiling
Gender Differences	Male testes descend from abdomen-----------------; Hearing development more acute in females; Male activity level greater

Reprinted with permission from Standley, J.M. (1998). Pre and perinatal growth and development: Implications of music benefits for premature infants. International Journal of Music Education, 31, 1-13.

Figure 1. Developmental Chart for Severely Premature Infants

Premature infant development between 24-40 weeks gestation age (GA) in neonatal intensive care follows virtually the same sequence of development as that of the fetus in the last trimester. Figure 1 illustrates the typical timeline by area of growth.

At 23-24 weeks, spontaneous and evoked fetal movements are fully developed. The infant turns its head, moves its hand to its head and face, and kicks, etc. He/she is beginning to respond to pain, though the response is somewhat slower than that of term infants. There are no social or interactive behaviors because the infant's limited resources are focused on survival and all responses are turned inwardly. The eyes are fused. Response to sound is inconsistent, though present, from 16 weeks. The taste and olfactory senses and preferences are functioning and developing. The survival rate of infants born at this gestational age is approximately 50%.

At 25-27 weeks, the eyes re-open and the infant begins to respond to light. There is a consistent startle response to sound. From 24-27 weeks the infant exhibits a single, unchanging behavioral state that is neither sleep nor wakefulness. Infants born at this gestational age have a survival rate of 80-90%. Some 10-25% of infants born at less than 28 weeks GA will leave the NICU with a pervasive developmental disability (PDD).

At 28 weeks, the testes in a male infant begin to descend from the abdomen. It is also theorized that neurological changes begin occurring due to the infusion of testosterone. Between 28 and 30 weeks, hearing is fully developed, but auditory thresholds are high. The lungs are capable of breathing air, though medical help may be needed. The infant will not be able to maintain body temperature, so placement on an open warmer or in an incubator will be necessary. The infant at this gestational age is skinny, has translucent skin and will lie with extended limbs. He/she is unable to curl into a fetal position without positioning assistance. At this birth age, survival is greater than 90%.

Between 31 and 33 weeks, the nerve pathways conveying pain responses finish myelinating. From this point forward, all skin receptors are functioning and there will be a full response to pain. The infant is usually breathing well enough to no longer need assistance from mechanical respiration and is ready to be "promoted" to intermediate care level within the NICU. He/she has begun organizing activity into discernible behavioral states. Visual acuity is still not fully developed and is poor, but visual focusing has begun. The infant begins to track horizontally and vertically. Suvival rate is 99%.

At 34 weeks, the suck-swallow-breathe coordinated response develops. Now the infant is ready to try feeding by mouth. At 34 weeks, the cartilage of the pinna develops in the ear and at 35 weeks, the auditory thresholds have decreased and are close to adult levels. Socially, the infant begins "coming out" and responding positively to caregivers and parents. At 35 weeks, the infant begins to engage in active sleep. At 36 weeks the infant can firmly grasp. At 37 weeks quiet sleep is possible.

During this period, the eyesight is improving and the infant can focus on brightly colored/contrasting objects about 10-12 inches away. The infant sees black, white, and red contrasts best. He/she can also lift the head for a brief moment. Infants with no further medical problems who are feeding well may be discharged during this period since they will usually thrive better in the home than in the medically-oriented NICU.

From 38-40 weeks, the infant is responding similarly to a full-term infant. At 38 weeks the infant begins visual and auditory orientation and tracking, though a head turn toward an auditory stimulus is delayed 8-11 seconds. Infants are now ready to bond with caregivers, reciprocate social interactions, and even smile in response to positive stimulation. Most infants are now ready to leave the hospital and go home. Their behavioral states will be similar to term infants and in about the same quantity throughout the 24-hour day: sleep (66%), drowsiness (8%), alertness (10%), fussiness (11%), and crying (5%). These "graduates" will also approximate term infants with regard to the following physiological ranges: heart rate of 120-160 beats/minute; respiratory rate of 30-60 inhalations/minute.

Developmental Intervention in the NICU

Assessment

Individualized care of premature infants using non-technological behavioral and nurturing interventions enhances neurological outcomes (Glass, 1994). The Assessment of Preterm Infants Behavior (APIB) (Als, Lester, Tronick, & Brazelton, 1982) evaluates the capabilities of the premature infant in the degree of smoothness and modulation, regulation, and differentiation of five behaviorally observable systems of functioning: autonomic, motor, state regulation, attentional/interactional, and self-regulatory. It identifies the infant's ability to interact with the environment and provides information for individualized and appropriate treatment and developmental interactions. The Brazelton Neonatal Behavioral Assessment Scale assesses similar functions for the healthy term infant and is commonly given to premature infants at discharge or shortly thereafter to monitor progress.

Treatment Planning

The NICU staff, including the Music Therapist, meets weekly in a patient care conference to determine treatment needs of each individual infant. Infant characteristics and progress are reported as are developing problems and plans for treatment. The NICU

Premature Infant Assessment and Treatment History

Birth History
Infant's name:________________ Gender: m f DOB___/___/___
Birthweight:____lb____oz/______k Gestational Age - Dubowitz______wks.
APGARs ___,___,___ Type Delivery: C-section Vaginal Breech Abruption

Family History
Mother's name________________________________ Age______ Gravita_____ Para_____
Father's name____________________________ Phone (H)_________ (W) __________
Address____
Occupations____
Related Issues____ Call/Visit
Admitting Diagnoses: meconium dusky HMD pneumonia hernias
genetic screen CP screen

Infant's Ongoing NICU Status
Date_______ Date_______ Date_______ Date_______
Age______days Age______days Age______days Age______days
AGA_____wks AGA_____wks AGA_____wks AGA_____wks
Wt________ Wt________ Wt________ Wt________

Bedding: Radiant warmer Incubator Open Crib Co-bedding
Respiration: No Assist. Ventilator CPAP Oxygen hood Nasal Cannula Room air
Nutrition: TPN/Lipids NPO G-tube OG/NG PO(bottle/breast) OG/PO PO
# of Weekly Apnea/Bradycardia Episodes: _______ _______ _______ _______

Medical Complications/Surgeries
UA/UVC Peripheral IV
Phototherapy
Medications:____
Intaventricular hemorrhage or Date of normal cranial ultrasound_______
PDA/murmur (Date of ligation______________)
Tested positive for: drugs HIV Staph Pseudomonas
Genetic abnormality __________________
Rickets
Tracheostomy
Necrotizing enterocolitis (Date of Colostomy_________)
Eye surgery
Hydrocephalus (Date of shunt ______________)
Other____

Referrals:
PT/OT: tonus/rigidity feeding problems calming rotation of extremities
MT: Continuous music for: ____ O2 Sat ____respiration stability at extubation
Multi-modal stimulation
PAL for:____ NNS _____feeding endurance
Parent training for overstimulation
Parent counseling
HS WIC CMS Home Monitoring Child and Family Services
Nesting date____________ Discharge date______________

Figure 2. Premature Infant Assessment and Treatment History Form

Abbreviations

APGAR APGAR test scores

CMS Children's Medical Services

CP cerebral palsy

CPAP continuous positive airway pressure

DOB date of birth

F female

G-tube gastrostomy device

HIV Human Immunodeficiency Virus

HMD hyaline membrane disease

HS Healthy Start Program

lb pound

m male

MT Music Therapy

No Assist. No respiratory assistance needed by infant

NNS non-nutritive sucking

NPO nothing by mouth

OG/NG oral or naso-gastric tube for feeding

O_2 Sat Oxygen saturation level

oz ounce

PAL Pacifier activated lullaby mechanism

PDA patent ductus arteriosus

PO by mouth, indicating breast or bottle feeding

PT/OT physical and/or occupational therapy for feeding, positioning, muscle development

Staph Staphyllococcus

TPN total parenteral nutrition

UA/UVC umbilical artery or venus catheter

WIC Women Infants Children food supplement program

Wks weeks

Form developed by Jennifer Whipple for use in Clinical Music Therapy Program at Tallahassee Memorial Hospital, 2001.

Figure 2 continued. Premature Infant Assessment and Treatment History Form

interdisciplinary team assesses basic developmental goals for each child during treatment and begins to establish general criteria which become prerequisites for discharge.

The Premature Infant Assessment and Treatment History form (Figure 2) provides a systematic way of recording individual infant progress across the entire NICU stay and medical, family, and developmental issues taken into account for treatment planning. The birth history section is the starting point and alerts one to potential problems for screening and assessment. The family history section relates to the parent's child development knowledge, resources, and time for infant care when discharge plans are made. Families with many children, those living far away from medical resources, and those with full-time work commitments often need additional assistance when taking a premature infant home. Those with other severe health or social problems may also require counseling.

The ongoing NICU status section assesses maturity and progress toward discharge. Medical complications and surgeries often disrupt or postpone developmental interventions. The referral section allows for coordinated services across disciplines. Community referrals are made for a smooth transition to home at hospital discharge. Nesting occurs prior to discharge and all parent training must be completed by that time. Discharge ends the treatment plan, though the infant may attend the NICU follow-up clinic as an outpatient or may be re-admitted as new problems develop. Readmission is usually made to the Pediatric Intensive Care Unit, not the NICU.

The NBICU Music Therapy Patient Information form (Figure 3) gives a complete picture of all infants in NICU care for a given week. It aids in planning delivery and allocation of treatment services and contains similar information to the previous form.

TMH NBICU/NBIMCU Music Therapy Patient Information

Date ____________________ HR I

MTref	Name	Family Info	Infant Info	Bed	Infant Status	Family Issues
MM PAL	new____ ______________ ______________ M / F Twin A / B Triplet A / B / C DOB__________ Dr.___________	Town __________________ Mother __________________ Age _______ Gr/Pa_________Ab_____ Father	_______dub Apg_________ Delivery= CS VD Br Abruption ______D __________W (CGA) ______Kg ______Lb ______oz complications:	OW I OC co-bed	O2= Vent ____% NC RA CPAP Hood Nutrition= G-tube OG PO____x/day TPN/L NPO PICC IV Fluids Cranial Ultra____________________ PhotoTherapy____ A/B's___ UA / UVC Meds:	Calls Visits Discharge date __________ by / on / after
MM PAL	new____ ______________ ______________ M / F Twin A / B Triplet A / B / C DOB__________ Dr.___________	Town __________________ Mother __________________ Age _______ Gr/Pa_________Ab_____ Father	_______dub Apg_________ Delivery= CS VD Br Abruption ______D __________W (CGA) ______Kg ______Lb ______oz complications:	OW I OC co-bed	O2= Vent ____% NC RA CPAP Hood Nutrition= G-tube OG PO____x/day TPN/L NPO PICC IV Fluids Cranial Ultra____________________ PhotoTherapy____ A/B's___ UA / UVC Meds:	Calls Visits Discharge date __________ by / on / after
MM PAL	new____ ______________ ______________ M / F Twin A / B Triplet A / B / C DOB__________ Dr.___________	Town __________________ Mother __________________ Age _______ Gr/Pa_________Ab_____ Father	_______dub Apg_________ Delivery= CS VD Br Abruption ______D __________W (CGA) ______Kg ______Lb ______oz complications:	OW I OC co-bed	O2= Vent ____% NC RA CPAP Hood Nutrition= G-tube OG PO____x/day TPN/L NPO PICC IV Fluids Cranial Ultra____________________ PhotoTherapy____ A/B's___ UA / UVC Meds:	Calls Visits Discharge date __________ by / on / after
MM PAL	new____ ______________ ______________ M / F Twin A / B Triplet A / B / C DOB__________ Dr.___________	Town __________________ Mother __________________ Age _______ Gr/Pa_________Ab_____ Father	_______dub Apg_________ Delivery= CS VD Br Abruption ______D __________W (CGA) ______Kg ______Lb ______oz complications:	OW I OC co-bed	O2= Vent ____% NC RA CPAP Hood Nutrition= G-tube OG PO____x/day TPN/L NPO PICC IV Fluids Cranial Ultra____________________ PhotoTherapy____ A/B's___ UA / UVC Meds:	Calls Visits Discharge date __________ by / on / after

Figure 3. TMH NBICU/NBIMCU Music Therapy Patient Information

Abbreviations by Column

Upper left information **Date** Date of the meeting
HR high risk infant status
I Intermediate infant status

MTref music therapy referral
MM music therapy multimodal stimulation
PAL pacifier activated lullaby mechanism

Name of infant
M male
F female
A/B twin designation of order of birth, A=first
A/B/C triplet designation of order of birth, A=first
DOB date of birth
Dr. physician

Family Info (information)
Gr/Pa gravita (# of pregnancies) and para (number of living children)
Ab abortion

Infant Info (information)
dub estimated gestational age by Dubowitz
Apg Apgar scores
CS Cesarean section
VD Vaginal delivery
Br Breech delivery
D days of age
W (CGA) age in weeks (corrected gestational age) i.e., Dubowitzage at delivery plus number of weeks of life.
Kg Lb oz current weight in kilograms or converted to pounds and ounces

Bed
OW open warmer also known as radiant warmer
I Incubator
OC open crib
co-bed co-bedding, i.e., twins or triplets placed in same bed

Infant Status
O2 oxygen
Vent ventilator
% per cent oxygen given
NC nasal canula
RA room air
CPAP continuous positive airway pressure
Hood oxygen hood
G-tube gastrostomy device
OG oral gastric tube
PO feeding by mouth
x/day times/day
TPN/L total parenteral nutrition and lipids
NPO nothing by mouth
PICC peripheral intravenous catheter
IV Fluids Fluids given by intravenous liine
Cranial Ultra cranial ultrasound
A/Bs number of apnea or bradycardia episodes for the week
UA /UVC Umbilical artery or venus catheter
Meds Medications

Form developed by Darcy Walworth for use in Tallahassee Memorial Hospital NICU MT program, 2002.

Figure 3 continued. TMH NBICU/NBIMCU Music Therapy Patient Information form

NICU Phases of Developmental Intervention

Research has just begun on the benefits versus limitations of early intervention programs occurring during the most critical phase of premature treatment in the NICU. Any music therapy programs designed for this phase of treatment must take into account the developmental responses at the premature level.

Survival/Pacification Phase. This phase occurs from very premature birth of 23-24 weeks up to approximately 30 gestational weeks. In addition to necessary medical treatment, a primary objective of the NICU is to pacify and soothe the very premature infant with all optional stimuli limited as much as possible. Even minimal stimuli are easily overwhelming to these neurologically immature patients, so lighting is reduced, sound levels are reduced, touching is restricted, swaddling and containment are usual, and medical procedures are grouped together to allow intervals of rest and recovery following intervention.

The infant may be placed in the fetal position or other position designed to facilitate specific muscle development. It is theorized that the close confinement of the womb in the final trimester allows the fetus to push against the mother's body, movement that is essential to infant muscle development. Containment or positioning in the NICU can approximate this critical womb development and eliminate atrophy from the child lying supine on a bed for an extended time. It also helps balance flexion and extension postures.

The nerve receptors in the skin are immature and hypersensitive. Light touch is particularly distressful to the very premature infant. Initially touch is allowed only for medical procedures. As the infant matures, the hand is placed in a stationary position on the infant's chest for warmth and security. Eventually, holding the swaddled infant for short periods and firm stroking will be tolerated.

The infant's lungs are immature and respiratory assistance is usually necessary prior to 32 weeks adjusted gestational age (AGA). The infant may be placed on a respirator and given oxygen with intermittent positive pressure ventilation (IPPV) or continuous positive airway pressure (CPAP). If a ventilator is not necessary, then oxygen may be delivered by hood or nasal canula. During this period, the infant will be monitored for apnea (absence of breathing) and bradycardia (absence of heart beat). Research has shown that listening to recorded lullabies improves infants' oxygen saturation levels during respiratory assistance (Cassidy & Standley, 1995; Standley & Moore, 1995) as does listening to the mother's voice and soothing sounds (Moore, Gladstone, & Standley, 1994).

Overwhelming stimuli and painful medical procedures create stress which releases cortisol leading to damaged neurological cell networks. Research shows that music listening reduces cortisol release in adults under stress (Standley, 2000b) and it may, therefore, have similar benefits for premature infants. We know that music calms infants and that very distressed NICU patients calm to music stimuli (Collins & Kuck, 1991). Caine (1992) and Chapman (1979) demonstrated that playing recorded music in the NICU increased infant weight gains. They speculated that calming results in less movement which saves calories and increases weight.

Initially, infants identify their mother by smell. Often a cloth with the mother's breast milk is placed in the incubator to comfort the premature infant and promote bonding with the mother. This can be paired with other comforting stimuli such as music to further enhance pacification. A lullaby sung and recorded by the mother and played frequently also becomes familiar and comforting, promotes bonding, and provides a familiar reference for the infant when the transition to the home environment is made.

Cautious Stimulation Phase. When an infant has achieved approximately 2.5 lbs. of weight and shows neurological maturity and readiness then, his/her developmental objectives can include cautious stimulation. The premature infant is hypersensitive to stimuli and all stimulation is cumulative. The younger the infant's gestational age, the more easily he/she is overwhelmed by stimuli. The initial indices of overstimulation include the following subtle disengagement cues: hiccoughs, grimace, clinched eyes, eyes averted, tongue protrusion, finger splay, or struggling movement. If these occur all stimulation should be stopped. After a pause of 15 seconds, then resumption of the interaction with just one stimulus may be attempted. Additional stimuli may be added slowly, one-at-a-time.

More potent disengagement cues consist of: crying, whining, fussing, cry face, spitting/vomiting, or hand in halt position. If these cues occur, again, all stimulation is stopped. The infant is placed back into the incubator and allowed to rest.

In all interactions, it is imperative to closely observe the infant's cues and control the interaction to avoid overstimulation. Faster habituation to stimulation equates to greater maturation and indicates that the infant is progressing developmentally (Kagan & Lewis, 1965). Unchanging music promotes homeostasis during other forms of stimulation and assists this habituation process.

Carefully controlled stimulation will alleviate some of the adverse neurological effects of preterm birth and negative consequences of prolonged hospitalization (Benes, 1994; Britt & Myers, 1994; Gomes-Pedro et al., 1995; Harrison, 1987; Oehler, 1993; White-Traut & Tubeszewski, 1986). Benefits from supplemental stimulation such as kangaroo care (skin to skin contact with the parent), massage, and music listening have been noted primarily in increased weight gain and improved motor development (Burns, Cunningham, White-Traut, Silvestri, & Nelson, 1994). Stroking promotes breathing in the neonate. Therefore, massage and kangaroo care are excellent therapies which can be paired with music when the infant is ready for multimodal stimulation (Standley, 1998).

Now, positioning with the hands accessible to the mouth allows the infant to explore, suck, and calm him/herself. Infants need opportunity for nonnutritive sucking. Sucking is the first rhythmic behavior in which the infant engages and it is theorized to contribute to neurological development by facilitating internally regulated rhythms (Goff, 1985). Extended time spent in non-nutritive sucking (NNS) has been observed to be a primary behavior of the third trimester fetus. It is theorized that NNS activates the vagus nerve which promotes the release of gastrointestinal hormones. These hormones stimulate secretory activity, growth of the GI tract, promotion of glucose-induced insulin release and enhancement of the infant's energy economy. Research has shown that non-nutritive sucking also increases oxygenation in the premature infant (Burroughs, Asonye, Anderson-Shanklin, & Vidyasagar, 1973). Music can be used to reinforce sucking rate and endurance (Standley, 2000a).

The coordinated suck/swallow/breathe ability develops around 34 weeks of gestation. Prior to that, premature infants are fed by tube. Clinical protocol recommends that pacifiers be paired with tube feedings to teach sucking with feeding sensations. Research has shown such non-nutritive sucking opportunities increase daily weight gain (Field et al., 1982).

Some infants must be taught to nipple feed after being tube fed for an extended period. Upon achieving 34 weeks gestation age, critically premature infants often need physical therapy to develop sustained feeding attention, seal capability, and sucking endurance strong enough to allow them to gain adequate daily nutrition by mouth. Contingent music has been shown to increase feeding rate (Standley, 2003).

Transition to Interactive Learning. This phase usually occurs around 32 weeks corrected gestational age. There is increasing concern that the strictures of life sustaining health care are detrimental to the preterm infant's prospects for intellectual development. Additionally, health care personnel have become concerned that almost all stimulation in this environment is both noncontingent and nonreciprocal and thus may have lifelong implications for decreased intellectual development (Burns et al., 1994). It is also known that incubator noise and ambient sounds in the NICU mask the frequencies of the human voice and may contribute to the premature infant's deprivation from normal auditory input (Glass, 1994).

After a full-term birth, infant learning normally occurs in an environment of reciprocal participation in cause/effect relationships and researchers feel this is a key element for normal brain development. When the infant cries, he/she is often picked up or, when hungry, is usually fed. Research has shown that one day after birth, term infants can respond to and demonstrate discrimination of a stimulus with a contingent reward (DeCasper & Carstens, 1981). However, in this same study the infants who first received the same stimulus noncontingently never learned the relationship between the contingent stimulus provided later and their behavior.

Presented with a contingent relationship, the term infant is capable of recognizing and responding to it very quickly. A study by Standley and Madsen (1990) not only revealed that babies as early as one month of age demonstrated awareness of the contingent relationship between their response and auditory stimulus onset, but learned the relationship within approximately 2.5 minutes.

In the NICU, interactions, feeding, and environmental changes seldom are presented contingently upon an infant "request" or cry. A medical schedule is the more likely determination of when an interaction occurs. Thus, prolonged treatment in this environment interferes with normal cause/effect or response contingent learning opportunities.

Providing structured learning opportunities while the premature infant remains in the medical environment is an evolving concept of developmental enhancement with little precedent in the research literature. However, there is a great deal of research that demonstrates music is an effective reinforcer for all ages of individuals achieving diverse behavior change in educational, home, and/or health care settings (Schunk, 1993; Standley, 1991, 1996).

A few studies have focused on music and infant learning. A meta-analysis on music as a reinforcer for infant learning in the first year of life demonstrated an overall Cohen's *d* effect size of 1.15 (Standley, 2001). The contingent music in the seven studies analyzed had a positive and significant impact on the treatment variables. Premature infants need opportunities to learn cause/effect relationships and music is an effective reinforcer, particularly lullabies sung by a female voice. It is known that term newborns attend more fixedly to music than to other auditory stimuli which may explain its reinforcement potential. There is also a great deal of evidence demonstrating the effectiveness of early childhood and infant stimulation music therapy techniques on developmental progress of at-risk children (Humpal, 2001a, 2001b).

Initial infant development goals involve awareness of environmental stimuli then demonstration of discriminations among different stimuli. Critical to this level of maturation is the ability for sustained awareness to the environment and changes within it. For instance the infant should orient to and track visual and auditory stimuli. This might be assisted by placing black and white and red objects, geometric designs, musical stimuli, and, eventually, interactive stimuli in the crib. Using guided assistance, the child is helped to manipulate objects or to turn the head toward the source of stimulation.

Music is a highly satisfactory input mode for the relay of information to the preterm infant. Language development is faster if the language is individually directed to the infant (rather than recorded) and if it is provided in "parentese" (speech with song-like qualities) (Trehub, Unyk, & Trainor, 1993). "Parentese," or the way adults tend to speak with babies is very similar to lullaby music and this seems to be a universal, cross-cultural similarity. Characteristics of "parentese" include extended vowels, mellifluous sounds, narrow pitch range rising for stimulation and falling for pacification, and repeated pitch contours. Lullabies sung by the mother or another female (the infant's preferred voices) can pacify and simultaneously promote language development.

Early intervention with music during the premature infant's NICU stay is still developing and long-term benefits are not yet documented by research. However, in existing NICU music therapy research, the usual benefits of the tested techniques have been earlier discharge from the NICU and evidence of increased developmental maturation upon discharge. This has positive implications for long-term benefits of exposure to music in the NICU.

Discharge

Discharge of the infant from the NICU encompasses both medical and non-medical family goals. Medical goals include the infant's ability to maintain body temperature in an open crib (usually around 34 weeks or 4.5 pounds) and to feed by mouth with a weight gain of almost an ounce/day (20-30 g). Additionally, the infant's need for oxygen and medication are stable and there is no need for hospital-managed medications. Non-medical goals include the parents' or caregivers' ability to manage the infant's physical and medical needs and to recognize problems that may require re-hospitalization.

Family Goals. The interdisciplinary team caring for the baby sets goals and provides pre-discharge training so that parents may learn to care for their infant's needs. During their NICU stay, families are gradually exposed to and taught to, care for, feed, and bathe their child. They must also learn the following critical skills.

- Family must learn to interpret and respond to infant signals while avoiding over-stimulation. Multimodal stimulation training assists parents with this objective (Whipple, 2000).
- Family must learn to care for infant's special needs. Some infants go home with life sustaining assistive devices: gastrointestinal tubes for feeding, oxygen and tracheostomy tubes for breathing, and/or heart rate and breathing monitors for apnea/bradycardia. The family members must learn to care for this equipment and their anxiety is great. Music therapy for anxiety reduction, guided imagery, and music for pleasure during this stressful time are important services.
- Family must learn importance and techniques of early intervention and developmental training for child. They must also learn to identify the emerging evidence of developmental delays that require intervention. They must also access and use early intervention programs to enhance development of the premature child.

Prior to discharge, the parents will probably "nest" with the child in the hospital. This is an opportunity for the parents to spend a few days and nights with the infant in the NICU area of the hospital and to be responsible for care of the infant. If problems arise, the NICU staff is immediately available for consultation. Parents usually need this interim level of responsibility prior to taking the infant home.

Follow-up Services. Specific family needs are determined during discharge planning and follow-up referrals made to allied therapies and community service agencies. Some home-based medical agencies provide monitors and other equipment, oxygen, parent training, and nursing services to premature infants discharged with special needs. The state Child and Family Services agency evaluates questionable home placements for infants due to violence, substance abuse, or child abuse and neglect and may arrange foster home placement. When necessary, custody of the child is given to Child and Family Services by the courts. Other infants are adopted immediately upon discharge from the NICU.

The NICU usually provides a follow-up clinic for infants with the greatest risk for developmental problems. These criteria include those with a birth weight less than 1500 grams, those with gestational age at birth less than 32 weeks, those who required more than 2 days on the ventilator, and those with neurological risk factors. These infants are invited to attend the clinic at intervals of 4 months corrected age, 1 year, 2 years, and 3 years.

WIC is a special food program for Women, Infants, and Children that is funded by the federal government. Eligible persons include a pregnant woman, a breastfeeding mother, a new mother, an infant, or a child up to 5 years of age. To qualify, these persons must be below an established income level and have a nutritional need that can be helped by WIC.

Many states offer special medical services to premature infants who qualify. In Florida, this agency is Children's Medical Services. The Children's Medical Services Program (CMS) provides a full range of medical services to children who are Medicaid eligible and who have special health care needs from birth to 21 years of age. These are children with serious or chronic physical or developmental conditions who require extensive preventive and maintenance care beyond that required by typically healthy children. Included are prevention and early intervention services, primary and specialty medical care, and long-term care for medically complex, fragile children. These funds can pay for the doctor, hospital costs, or home health care.

In Florida, prenatal and perinatal services are provided to improve birth outcomes. By state legislation signed in 1991, the Healthy Start program provides prenatal and perinatal screening, referral, and care coordination services. Pregnant women are screened for risk factors such as history of smoking or alcohol/drug use, marital status, and race. Infants are screened for low birth weight status and exposure to toxins during fetal development.

The Early Intervention Program (EIP) is a pre-kindergarten learning opportunity funded through federal IDEA program legislation. It is for economically disadvantaged children aged 3-4 years and others of the same age who are at risk of future school failure.

References

Als, H., Lester, B., Tronick, E., & Brazelton, T. (1982). Manual for the assessment of preterm infants' behavior (APIB). In H. Fitzgerald, B. Lester, & M. Yogman (Eds.), *Theory and research in behavioral pediatrics* (pp. 65-132). New York: Plenum Press.

American Academy of Pediatrics. Committee on Environmental Health. (1997). Noise: A hazard for the fetus and newborn. *Pediatrics*, 100(4), 724-727.

Benes, F. M. (1994). Development of the corticolimbic system. In G. Dawson & K. Gischer (Eds.), *Human behavior and the developing brain* (pp. 176-206). New York: Guilford Press.

Britt, G., & Myers, B. (1994). The effects of Brazelton intervention: A review. *Infant Mental Health*, 15(3), 278-292.

Burns, K., Cunningham, N., White-Traut, R., Silvestri, J., & Nelson, M. (1994). Infant stimulation: Modification of an intervention based on physiologic and behavioral cues. *Journal of Obstetric, Gynecologic, and Neonatal Nursing*, 23(7), 581-589.

Burroughs, A., Asonye, U., Anderson-Shanklin, G., & Vidyasagar, D. (1973). The effect of nonnutritive sucking on transcutaneous oxygen tension in noncrying, preterm neonates. *Research in Nursing and Health*, 1(2), 69-75.

Caine, J. (1992). The effects of music on the selected stress behaviors, weight, caloric and formula intake, and length of hospital stay of premature and low birth weight neonates in a newborn intensive care unit. *Journal of Music Therapy*, 28(4), 180-192.

Cassidy, J., & Ditty, K. (2001). Gender differences among newborns on a transient otoacoustic emissions test for hearing. *Journal of Music Therapy*, 38(1), 28-35.

Cassidy, J. W., & Standley, J. M. (1995). The effect of music listening on physiological responses of premature infants in the NICU. *Journal of Music Therapy*, 32(4), 208-227.

Centers for Disease Control. (1999, April 29). *National Vital Statistics Report*, 47(18).

Chapman, J. S. (1979). Influence of varied stimuli on development of motor patterns in the premature infant. In G. Anderson & B. Raff (Eds.), *Newborn behavioral organization: Nursing research and implications* (pp. 61-80). New York: Alan Liss.

Cheour-Luhtanen, M., Alho, K., Sainio, K., Rinne, T., Reinikainen, K., Pohjavuouri, M., Renlund, M., Aaltonen, O., Eerola, O., & Naatanen, R. (1996). The ontogenetically earliest discriminative response of the human brain. *Psychophysiology*, 33, 478-481.

Chiron, C., Jambaque, I., Nabbout, R., Lounes, R., Syrota, A., & Dulac, O. (1997). The right brain hemisphere is dominant in human infants. *Brain*, 120(6), 1057-1065.

Collins, S. K., & Kuck, K. (1991). Music therapy in the Neonatal Intensive Care Unit. *Neonatal Network*, 9(6), 23-26.

Creasey, G., Jarvis, P., Myers, B., Markowitz, P., & Kerkering, K. (1993). Mental and motor development for three groups of premature infants. *Infant Behavior and Development*, 16, 365-372.

DeCasper, A. J., & Carstens, A. A. (1981). Contingencies of stimulation: Effects on learning and emotion in neonates. *Infant Behavior and Development*, 4(1), 19-35.

DeCasper, A. J., & Fifer, W. P. (1980). Of human bonding: Newborns prefer their mothers' voices. *Science*, 208, 1174-1176.

DeCasper, A. J., & Spence, M. J. (1986). Newborns prefer a familiar story over an unfamiliar one. *Infant Behavior and Development*, 9, 133-150.

Field, T., Ignatoff, E., Stringer, S., Brennan, J., Greenberg, R., Widmayer, S., & Anderson, G. (1982). Nonnutritive sucking during tube feedings: Effects on preterm neonates in an intensive care unit. *Pediatrics*, 70(3), 381-384.

Fischer, K. W., & Rose, S. T. (1994). Dynamic development of coordination of components in brain and behavior: A framework for theory and research. In G. Dawson & K. W. Fischer (Eds.), *Human behavior and the developing brain* (pp. 3-66). New York: Guilford Press.

Garcia-Prats, J. A. & Hornfischer, S. S. (2000). *What to do when your baby is premature.* New York: Three Rivers Press.

Glass, P. (1994). The vulnerable neonate and the neonatal intensive care environment. In G. B. Avery, M. A. Fletcher, & M. G. MacDonald (Eds.), *Neonatology: Pathophysiology and management of the newborn* (4th ed.; pp. 77-94). Philadelphia: J. B. Lippincott.

Goff, D. M. (1985). The effects of nonnutritive sucking on state regulation in preterm infants. *Dissertation Abstracts International*, 46, 08B-2835.

Gomes-Pedro, J., Patricio, M., Carvalho, A., Goldschmidt, T., Torgal-Garcia, F., & Monteiro, M. (1995). Early intervention with Portuguese mothers: A 2-year follow-up. *Journal of Developmental and Behavioral Pediatrics*, 16(1), 21-28.

Hack, M., Klein, N., & Taylor, H. (1995). Long-term developmental outcomes of low birth weight infants. *The Future of Children* [On-line serial], 5(1). Available: http://www.futureofchildren.org/LBW/12LBWHAC.htm.

Harrison, L. (1987). Effects of early supplemental stimulation programs for premature infants: Review of the literature. *Maternal-Child Nursing Journal*, 14(2), 69-90.

Horbar, J., & Lucey, J. (1995). Evaluation of neonatal intensive care technologies. *The Future of Children* [On-line serial], 5(1). Available: http://www.futureofchildren.org/ LBW/ 12LBWHAC.htm.

Humpal, M. (2001a). Annotated bibliography of music therapy articles related to young children: From music therapy journals (1990-2000). *Early Childhood Connections*, 7(2), 16-17.

Humpal, M. (2001b). Music therapy and the young child. *Early Childhood Connections*, 7(2), 9-15.

Inder, T., Huppi, P., Zientara, G., Maier, S., Jolesz, F., di Slavo, D., Robertson, R., Barnes, P., & Volpe, J. (1999). Early detection of peri leukomalacia by diffusion-weighted magnetic resonance imaging techniques. *Journal of Pediatrics*, 134(5), 631-634.

Johnston, C., Sherrard, A., Stevens, B., Franck, L., Stemler, R., & Jack, A. (1999). Do cry features reflect pain intensity in preterm neonates? A preliminary study. *Biology of the Neonate*, 76(2), 120-124.

Kagan, J., & Lewis, M. (1965). Studies of attention in the human infant. *Merrill-Palmer Quarterly*, 11, 95-127.

Karmel, B., Gardner, J., & Magnano, C. (1991). Attention and arousal in early infancy. In M. Weiss & P. Zelazo (Eds.). *Newborn attention: Biological constraints and the influence of experience* (pp. 339-376). Norwood, NJ: Ablex.

Klaus, M. H., & Fanaroff, A. A. (1993). *Care of the high risk infant*. Philadelphia: W. B. Saunders.

Kolata, G. (1984). Studying learning in the womb. *Science*, 225(4659), 302-303.

Kotulak, R. (1993). Unlocking the mind, a prize-winning series from the Chicago Tribune. *Chicago Tribune*, April, 1993.

Lecanuet, J., Granier-Deferre, C., & Busnel, M. (1995). Human fetal auditory perception. In J. P. Lecanuet, W. P. Fifer, N. A. Krasnegor, & W. P. Smotherman, (Eds.). *Fetal development: A psychobiological perspective* (pp. 239-262). Hillsdale, NJ: Lawrence Erlbaum.

Lewit, E., Baker, L., Corman, H., & Shiono, P. (1995). The direct cost of low birth weight. *The Future of Children* [On-line serial], 5(1). Available: http://www.futureofchildren.org/LBW/12LBWHAC.htm.

Maalouf, E., Duggan, P., Rutherford, M., Counsell, S., Fletcher, A., Battin, M., Cowan, F., & Edwards, A. (1999). Magnetic resonance imaging of the brain in a cohort of extremely preterm infants. *Journal of Pediatrics*, 135(3), 351-357.

Martin, J., Hamilton,, B., Ventura, S., Menacker, F., & Park, M. (2002, February 12). Births: Final data for 2000. *National Vital Statistics Reports*, 50(5).

Michel, P. (1973). The optimum development of musical abilities in the infant years of life. *Psychology of Music*, 1(2), 14-20.

Moog, H. (1976). *The musical experience of the preschool child.* London: Schott.

Moon, C., Cooper, R. P., & Fifer, W. P. (1993). Two-day-olds prefer their native language. *Infant Behavior and Development*, 16, 495-500.

Moore, R., Gladstone, I., & Standley, J. (1994). *Effects of music, maternal voice, intrauterine sounds and white noise on the oxygen saturation levels of premature infants.* Paper presented at the National Association for Music Therapy, Inc., National Conference, Orlando, FL.

Muir, D. W. (1985). The development of infants' auditory spatial sensitivity. In S. E. Trehub & B. A. Schneider (Eds.), *Auditory development in infancy* (pp. 55-83). New York: Plenum.

Oehler, J. (1993). Developmental care of low birth weight infants. *Advances in Clinical Nursing Research*, 28(2), 289-301.

Peterson, B., Vohr, B., Staib, L., Cannistraci, C., Dolber, A., Schneider, K., Katz, K., Westerveld, M., Sparrow, S., Anderson, A., Duncan, C., Makuch, R., Gore, J., & Ment, L. (2000). Regional brain volume abnormalities and long-term cognitive outcome in preterm infants. *Journal of the American Medical Association*, 284(15), 1939-1947.

Polverini-Rey, R. (1992). Intrauterine musical learning: The soothing effect on newborns of a lullaby learned prenatally. *Dissertation Abstracts International*, 53, 10A-3481.

Ries, N. L. (1982). An analysis of the characteristics of infant-child singing expressions. *Dissertation Abstracts International*, 43, 06A-1871.

Roeser, R. J. (1996), *Audiology desk reference.* New York: Thieme.

Roush, W. (1997). A womb with a view. *Science*, 278, 1397-1399.

Schunk, H. A. (1993). *The relationship between background music during feeding time and weight gain of low-birthweight infants: A pilot study.* Unpublished study presented at National Association for Music Therapy, Inc., National Conference, Toronto, Canada.

Shetler, D. (1989). The inquiry into prenatal musical experience: A report of the Eastman Project 1980-1987. *Pre- and Peri-Natal Psychology*, 3(3), 171-189.

Spitzer, A. R. (1996). *Intensive care of the fetus and neonate.* Baltimore: Mosby-Year Book.

Standley, J. (1991). The role of music in pacification/stimulation of premature infants with low birthweights. *Music Therapy Perspectives*, 9(1), 19-25.

Standley, J. (1996). A meta-analysis on the effects of music as reinforcement for education/therapy objectives. *Journal of Research in Music Education*, 44(2), 105-133.

Standley, J. (1998). The effect of music and multimodal stimulation on physiologic and developmental responses of premature infants in neonatal intensive care. *Pediatric Nursing*, 21(6), 532-539.

Standley, J. (2000a). The effect of contingent music to increase non-nutritive sucking of premature infants. *Pediatric Nursing*, 26(5), 493-495, 498-499.

Standley, J. (2000b). Music research in medical/dental treatment: An update of a prior meta-analysis. In American Music Therapy Association (Ed.), *Effectiveness of music therapy procedures: Documentation of research and clinical practice* (3rd ed.; pp. 1-60). Silver Spring, MD: American Music Therapy Association.

Standley, J. (2001). The power of contingent music for infant learning. *Bulletin of the Council for Research in Music Education*, No. 149, Spring, 65-71.

Standley, J. (2003). The effect of music-reinforced non-nutritive sucking on feeding rate of premature infants. *Journal of Pediatric Nursing*, 18(3), 169-173.

Standley, J., & Madsen, C. (1990). Comparison of infant preferences and responses to auditory stimuli: Music, mother, and other female voice. *Journal of Music Therapy*, 27(2), 54-97.

Standley, J., & Moore, R. (1995). Therapeutic effects of music and mother's voice on premature infants. *Pediatric Nursing*, 21(6), 509-512, 574.

Summers, E. K. (1984). Categorization and conservation of melody in infants. *Dissertation Abstracts International*, 45, 11B-3643-3644.

Tims, F. (1978). Contrasting music conditions, visual attending behavior and state in eight-week-old infants. *Dissertation Abstracts International*, 39, 07A-4111.

Tracy, A. E., & Maroney, D. I. (1999). *Your premature baby and child.* New York: Berkley.

Trehub, S. E., Unyk, A., & Trainor, L. (1993). Adults identify infant-directed music across cultures. *Infant Behavior and Development*, 16(2), 193-211.

Watt, T. J. (1994). Intraventricular hemorrhage in the premature infant. *Nebraska Medical Journal*, 79, 322-325

Wendrich, K. A. (1981). Pitch imitation in infancy and early childhood: Observations and implications. *Dissertation Abstracts International*, 41, 12A-5019.

Whipple, J. (2000). The effect of parent training in music and multimodal stimulation on parent-neonate interactions in the Neonatal Intensive Care Unit. *Journal of Music Therapy*, 37(4), 250-268.

White-Traut, R. C., & Tubeszewski, K. A. (1986). Multimodal stimulation of the premature infant. *Journal of Pediatric Nursing*, 1(2), 90-95.

Woodward, S., Guidozzi, F., Hofmeyr, G., De Jong, P., Anthony, J., & Woods, D. (1992). Discoveries in the fetal and neonatal worlds of music. In H. Lees (Ed.), *Music education: Sharing musics of the world* (pp. 58-66). Proceedings of the 20th World Conference of the International Society for Music Education, Seoul, Korea.

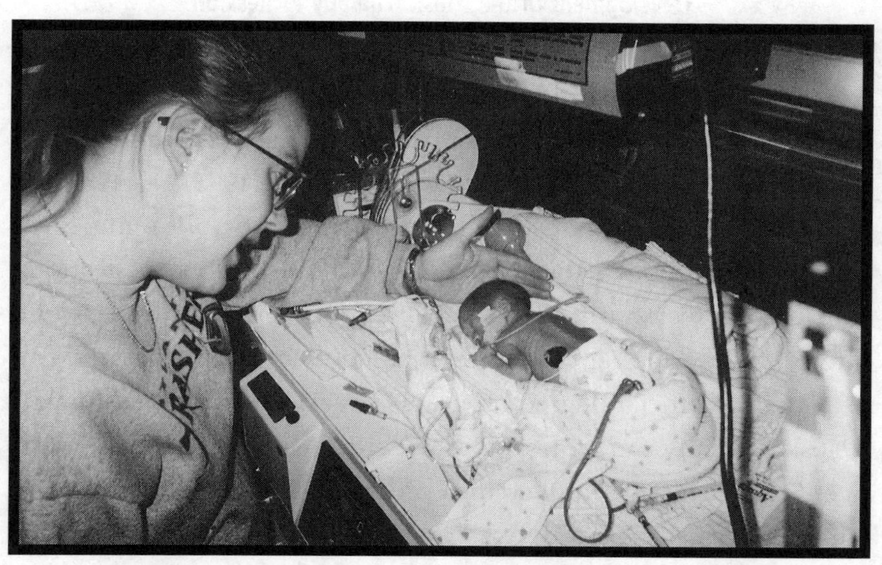

Libby is off the ventilator and making progress. She is ready for cautious touch and soothing verbal interactions with Mom. Quiet lullaby singing to promote homeostasis is recommended.

2 | Medical Music Therapy

Development of the Music Therapy Profession

Most historians attribute the beginning of the music therapy career in the United States to volunteer musicians giving concerts in Veterans Hospitals for traumatized soldiers immediately following World War II (Davis, Gfeller, & Thaut, 1992). Staff noticed that therapeutic changes occurred during and following these concerts and reported this in Veterans Administration publications. Music volunteerism in mental health programs increased, as did interest in developing professional practices in music therapy.

The first official degree programs began in America in the late 1940s. Currently, the profession is widely developed in the U.S. with over 70 colleges and universities providing degree programs. The American Music Therapy Association with almost 4,000 members suggests curricular guidelines and credentials for degrees at the bachelor's, master's, and doctoral levels.

A qualified music therapist completes at least a bachelor's degree which includes an internship in a clinical music therapy program of at least 1,200 hours. Upon completion of the undergraduate degree, the music therapist may then take a national exam to become Board Certified. A master's degree in music therapy is often sought for clinical specialization, while a doctorate is desirable for college teaching in this field.

The overall premise for the profession of music therapy is to achieve beneficial change in an individual or group through special music techniques. Music therapy treatment is based on identification of a specific problem; an assessment of problem severity and complexity; assessment of music preferences; a treatment plan with research-based music therapy techniques matched to the clients' problems, personality, and preferences; and systematic evaluation of results. The complete process is fully documented in the client's program record.

Music therapy combines knowledge of the human responses to music with principles of psychology, education, medicine, and rehabilitation. Music therapy techniques include the full gamut of human interactions with, and thoughts about, music: playing, singing, discussing, moving to, and composing or creating music (Standley, 2002a). People of all ages respond to music therapeutically and the individual's preference for type of music is very important to its therapeutic benefit. To be optimally effective for the widest range of people, the music therapist, therefore, combines classical music training with functional knowledge of music from many tastes and cultures.

National Organizations

The American Music Therapy Association (AMTA) is the nation's professional organization for the field of music therapy with a membership approaching 4,000. The AMTA resulted from the January 1, 1998 unification of the former National Association for Music Therapy, Inc. and the former American Association for Music Therapy. The AMTA currently approves the curriculum and faculty qualifications for music therapy degree programs for approximately 70 colleges and universities in the U.S. The address is: Dr. Andrea Farbman, Executive Director; American Music Therapy Association; 8455 Colesville Road, Suite 1000, Silver Spring, MD 20910; (301) 589-

3300, Fax: (301) 589-5175. The web addresses are info@musictherapy.org or www.musictherapy.org.

The Certification Board for Music Therapists is a separate and independent organization providing a national certification test to assist the public in identifying standards for the professional practice of music therapy. Persons who pass this test use the designation MT-BC, Music Therapist, Board Certified. The address for this organization is: Joy Scheck, Executive Director, Certification Board for Music Therapists, 506 East Lancaster Avenue, Suite 102, Downington, PA 19335; (800) 765-CBMT. The web address is www.cbmt.org.

Development and Rationale for Medical Music Therapy

Throughout history, healers have recorded anecdotes about the benefits of using music during medical treatment. Methodical study of this phenomenon began at the end of the 19th century and has resulted in development of a contemporary professional specialty, the medical music therapist. Research and clinical practice in medical treatment have shown that music therapy techniques reduce perception of pain, reduce stress, benefit psychological adjustment to trauma, and reduce stimulus deprivation during serious or extended illnesses. And unlike most medical treatments or medications, music has few, if any, unwanted side effects.

Unique Properties of Music

Music is acoustically different from all other sound and has valid and excellent therapeutic potential, especially in medical treatment. Sounds are caused by vibration and exist on a variety of continua: high/low, loud/soft, and diverse timbres and envelopes (Wagner, 1994). The envelope or temporal shape of a sound involves the progressive changes of the tone from moment to moment that help us identify one sound from another. These changes also serve to elicit our sustained attention across time.

Very few sounds are pure tones, the sound heard at a single frequency. Complex vibrations produce harmonics, the overtones whose frequencies are multiples of that of the original sound. All musical instruments and the human voice produce sounds with harmonics. Music in each culture is composed according to historically developed principles which have selected those sounds that are most pleasant, or "musical" to the human ear. Music is complex sound that is intellectually stimulating and pleasing to the senses.

Masking is the effect of one set of sounds impinging upon the perception of another set of sounds. Music, a pleasant set of sounds, is sometimes used to mask aversive auditory stimuli. Attention to pleasurable sound causes aversive sound to recede from perception.

Noise is sound with no fixed pitch. It is inconsistent vibration (to and fro motion without regular frequency) which contains inharmonic overtones. Inharmonic overtones have inconsistencies of tension, stress and configuration which bring fatigue and stress to the listener. Ambient sound is the composite of the noises in one's environment. Too much ambient sound produces irritation. By contrast, its total absence is disconcerting (Wagner, 1994).

Aural perception is a neurological ability to perceive and translate the vibrations to which we are exposed. It must be developed as we neurologically mature from fetal to adult state. The temporal lobes of the brain receive auditory signals from the inner ear through many different routes. For instance, neurons in one path respond to high tones, while those along a different path respond to low tones. These pathways must be established in conjunction with their associated translation, including differentiation, recognition, and memory of individual sounds. This allows us to have perfect pitch, recognize the trumpet or a birdcall from all other sounds, and reproduce the melody to "Twinkle, Twinkle, Little Star" that we learned as a child.

Music has many cognitive elements: melody, rhythm, harmony, timbre, form style, and expressive nuances (Farnsworth, 1958). These are processed simultaneously or sequentially while listening to music. The same two notes sound, and are perceived, very differently when played sequentially versus simultaneously.

Melodies are successive intervals (distance between notes) with organization. We learn the organization through repeated listening; we then develop expectancies about the way that intervals will be heard in future occurrences. These expectancies and perception of their appearance seem to be a very pleasing activity of the brain. The tempo or speed of the melody may be an index of its function on our perception and subsequent emotions.

The neurological response to tonal stimuli is to try to determine vibration ratios and make "sense" or "order" of them. Dissonances will fatigue a listener sooner than consonances. It is theorized that the brain enjoys this process of "ordering" sound until fatigue sets in. Therefore, music is more pleasant, soothing, interesting, etc., than noise (Wagner, 1994).

There is no piece of music that can be consistently labeled stimulative or sedative. Rather, research shows this is a learned perception of the listener. For instance, some teens sleep to their "sedative music," punk rock, which their parents perceive as highly stimulating, even irritating. In order to predict that a piece of music will sedate or stimulate a particular individual, that person's history with that musical selection must be taken into account.

The brain also stores music according to emotional content and association. Upon hearing the musical selection, the emotion associated with it is also activated. This is a powerful aspect of music's attraction to all humans. Each person's culture, learning experiences, emotional development, and individual preferences are very important aspects in selection of music in therapy.

Research in Music and Medical Treatment

Medical music therapy is a relatively new profession, but very ancient idea and practice. Throughout written history music has been associated with the treatment of disease. The Kahum papyrus is the oldest known written account of medical practices and refers to the use of incantations for healing the sick (Light, Love, Benson, & Morch, 1954). At the end of the 19th century, physicians began a transition from anecdotal to research evidence concerning music. Their early studies showed beneficial effects of music on specific physiological processes such as cardiac output, respiratory rate, pulse rate, and blood pressure (Light et al., 1954).

Taylor's history of music in general hospital treatment (1981) credits Evan O'Neill Kane with the initial clinical use of music during surgery. In 1914, his creative use of a phonograph in the operating room calmed patients prior to the application of anesthesia. Many patients find the anxiety about a medical procedure to be more debilitating than the procedure itself. Since this initial study, music's effects on stress and anxiety have been exhaustively researched (Hanser, 1985).

What can music add to other forms of medical treatment? After more than 100 years of study on this topic, a body of information now exists to document the many medical, social, and emotional benefits of music. A meta-analysis synthesizes a body of research and allows generalization for clinical program development. A meta-analysis of medical research showed that the overall, mean effect of music as measured by designated primary dependent variables was 1.17 (Standley, 2000b). This means that the average therapeutic effect of music in medical treatment was more than one standard deviation greater than that same treatment without music.

Table 2 shows a summary of the generalized effects of music that were derived from the above meta-analysis. Overall, it can be ascertained that women respond to music with greater effect than do men. By age, infants show the least effects.

Table 2. Meta-Analysis Results: Generalizations From the Research Literature About the Use of Music in Medical Treatment[1]

Gender	Women (ES=.90, *n*=30) respond to music with greater effect than do men (ES=.57, *n*=14). These data were based on studies utilizing subjects of only one gender group.
Age	Children and adolescents (ES=.95, *n*=26) respond with somewhat greater effect than do adults (ES=.87, *n*=158). Infants show the least response to music (ES=.48, *n*=34).
Pain	Music has slightly greater effect when some pain is present (ES=.87, *n*=193) than when it is not a usual symptom of the diagnosis (ES=.81, *n*=22), though music seems to become less effective as the pain increases.
Type Dependent Measures	The least conservative measure of music's effect is patient self-report (ES=.93, *n*=86) while systematic behavioral observation (ES=.83, *n*=50) and physiological measures (ES=.90, *n*=96) result in similar, but slightly more conservative effect sizes. The most frequently utilized dependent variable is a physiological measure.
Diagnoses	Effects vary widely according to diagnosis. Music seems to be less effective when severe pain is a usual symptom or the diagnosis has serious implications. Effects are greatest for dental patients and those with chronic pain, i.e., migraine headaches. More minimal effects are reported for obstetrical, burn, coma and cancer patients with lowest effects being reported for neonates and for use of music in the emergency room for laceration repair.
Music	Live music presented by a trained music therapist (ES=1.13, *n*=16) has a much greater effect than does recorded music (ES=.82, *n*=216). Preferred music has the greatest effect (ES=1.40, *n*=30).
Dependent Measures	Effects vary greatly according to the specific dependent measure utilized. Greatest effects were reported for grasp strength of stroke patients and perceived effectiveness of the music. Least effects were measured by days of hospitalization, peripheral finger temperature, ease of childbirth, time of recovery from anesthesia, formula intake of neonates and neonate apnea.

[1]Reprinted with permission from Standley, J.M. (2000b). Music research in medical/dental treatment: An update of a prior meta-analysis. In American Music Therapy Association (Ed.), *Effectiveness of music therapy procedures: Documentation of research and clinical practice* (3rd ed., pp. 1-60). Silver Spring, MD: American Music Therapy Association

It is also apparent that music's effects are greatest when the patient is experiencing some pain, but these effects are reduced as the pain becomes severe. Music is an established and effective audioanalgesic and is often used in therapy for pain management (Bailey, 1986; Corah, Gale, Pace, & Seyrek, 1981). Music therapists currently theorize that listening to auditory stimuli may directly suppress pain neurologically, or, alternatively, that focus on music may serve as a distraction from aversive stimuli to which patients have conditioned anxiety.

Finally, Table 2 shows that live music presented by a music therapist is far more powerful than is the use of recorded music. Live music has the benefits of being interactive with the patient and immediately being adapted by the music therapist to the ongoing, changing needs of the patient. Studies utilizing patients' preferred music demonstrated the greatest effect (ES=1.40, *n*=30).

As is true with most medical treatments, the table also demonstrates that the effects of music seem greatly differentiated according to patient diagnosis and related level of pain, anxiety, and prognosis. Neonates in need of medical services are shown to have the least effects of music. This is related to their early developmental stage which is neurologically and musically immature.

It should be noted that results of the above meta-analysis do not include any effects of musician-provided concerts in hospitals, a volunteer activity that has not been subjected to research investigation. Music in medicine programs are generally deemed to enhance the hospital environment and add pleasure to the patients' stay. These programs are separate and distinct from the music therapy profession and research-based treatment.

Medical Music Therapy With Children

In recent years, clinical music therapy programs have been developed for hospital pediatric units with procedures derived from the research literature (Brodsky, 1989; Cohen, 1984). There are many references to the benefits of music activities in reducing fear, distress, and anxiety of hospitalized infants, toddlers, and their families (Fagen, 1982; Hoffman, 1980; Lindsay, 1981; Marley, 1984; McDonnell, 1984; Miller, 1984; Robinson, 1962; Schwankovsky & Guthrie, 1982). Music therapy also helps children feel free to verbalize about the trauma of hospitalization (Froelich, 1984) and promotes creative "wellness" attributes and subsequent activities in the very ill child.

For infants, music can generally reduce crying (Lininger, 1987) even the prolonged and frequent crying of infants with colic (Larson & Ayllon, 1990). Pediatric patients exhibit reduced anxiety when listening to music during painful procedures such as cardiac catheterization (Caire & Erickson, 1986; Gettel, 1985; Micci, 1984). They also exhibit reduced fear during injections (Fowler-Kerry & Lander, 1987), intravenous starts and venipunctures (Malone, 1996), bone marrow aspirations (Pfaff, Smith, & Gowan, 1989), lumbar punctures (Rasco, 1992), and other painful pediatric oncology procedures (Lane, 1991; Standley & Hanser, 1994). Music therapy has also been shown to reduce respiratory distress (Ammon, 1968), preoperative anxiety (Aldridge, 1993; Chetta, 1981; Robb, Nichols, Rutan, Bishop, & Parker, 1995), and general pain (Clinton, 1984; Rudenberg & Royka, 1989; Schneider, 1982; Siegel, 1983; Steinke, 1991) in children. Music singing has even been used to reduce cystic fibrosis congestion (Kamps, 1992).

There are notable studies with clinically important results for premature infants. Chapman (1975) demonstrated the effects of lullabies in the neonatal nursery on weight gain and pacification of newborns. She combined music with motion and found a 16% reduction for premature infants in total time to reach weight criterion for discharge. Similar research studies with diverse dependent variables have shown that premature neonates benefit from listening to music while in the intensive care isolette (Katz, 1971). These babies demonstrate more stable physiological measures (Lorch, Lorch, Diefendorf, & Earl, 1994), show improved oxygen saturation levels (Cassidy & Standley, 1995; Coleman, Pratt, Stoddard, Gerstmann, & Abel, 1997; Collins & Kuck, 1991; Flowers, McCain, & Hilker, 1999; Moore, Gladstone, & Standley, 1994; Standley & Moore, 1995), increase their weight gain (Malloy, 1979), and are discharged sooner (Caine, 1991). Music has been shown to reduce distress following stressful procedures such as suctioning of premature infants on continuous ventilatory support (Burke, Walsh, Oehler, & Gingras, 1995). This happens every few hours, interrupts the infant's period of restful sleep, and causes distress.

A meta-analysis on music research with premature infants in NICUs was conducted and showed an overall large, significant, consistent effect size of almost a standard deviation (Cohen's d=.83) (Standley, 2002b). Table 3 shows that effects were not mediated by birth weight, gestational age at the time of study, or type of music delivery. All infants of all ages and birth weights benefited equally. Effects were not differentiated among physiological, behavioral, or developmental measures of benefit. This homogeneity of findings suggests that the addition of music to NICU care and developmental intervention provides both statistically significant and clinically important benefits.

Infant neurological development occurs during quiet sleep. Thus pacification technques have implication for enhanced development. Music with multimodal stimulation increases infant pacification and enhances developmental milestones. When mothers learn this approach, it has also enhances mother-infant bonding (Standley, 1991b, 1998; Whipple, 2000).

This pacification effect of music is the only one documented with long-term effects for premature infants. Infants from Caine's study who received music in the Neonatal Intensive Care Unit (NICU) were rated by their mothers at 6 months of age to be calmer than those without music intervention (Standley, 1991a).

Opportunities for cause/effect learning for hospitalized infants are critical. Standley has demonstrated that music is an effective contingency for increasing non-nutritive sucking of premature

Table 3. Characteristics of NICU Music Studies

Study	*n*	Independent Variable	Music Type/ Delivery	dB Level[1]	Adjusted Gestational Age @ Study[2]	Dependent Variable	Effect size Cohen's *d*
Caine, 1991	52	Lullabies vs. RAS[3]	Recorded/Free field	70-80	NA	Days in hospital	.51
						Weight gain	.84
						Behavior state	.73
Cassidy & Standley, 1998	20	Lullabies vs. RAS	Recorded/Earcups	80	27 wks.	Oxygen saturation	1.19
Coleman et al., 1997	66	Lullabies vs. RAS	Recorded/Free field	65-75	29.5 wks.	Heart rate	.91
						Oxygen saturation	.86
						Behavior state	1.95
						Days in hospital	.49
						Weight gain	.49
Collins & Kuck, 1996	17	Lullabies with heart beats	Recorded/Free field	80	30 wks.	Oxygen saturation	.70
						Behavior state	1.26
						Heart rate	.46
Flowers, 1999	9	'70s Ballads and lullabies with heart beats	Recorded/Free field	55	28 wks.	Oxygen saturation	1.05
						Behavior state	.88
Moore, Gladstone, & Standley, 1997	22	Lullabies vs. white noise	Recorded/Earphones	75-80	31 wks.	Oxygen saturation	1.29
Standley, 1998	40	Lullabies with Massage vs. RAS	Live singing	quiet	30.6 wks.	Days in hospital	.55
						Weight gain	.81
Standley, 2000a	12	Contingent lullabies for sucking	Recorded/Free field	65-70	35.5 wks	Non-nutritive sucking rate	.73
Standley, 2003	32	Lullabies contingent upon pacifier suck	Recorded/Free field	65-70	36.1 wks.	Feeding rate	.87
Standley & Moore, 1995	20	Lullabies vs. RAS	Recorded/Earphones	65-70	NA	Oxygen saturation	1.03

[1]It is unclear whether dB levels were determined with Scale A or Scale C measurements.
[2]Mean group age
[3]Routine Auditory Stimulation

Data reprinted with permission of *Journal of Pediatric Nursing* (Standley, 2002b).

infants (2000a) which also improves subsequent feeding ability (2003).

Medical Music Therapy Clinical Programs

A medical music therapy program is normally established in a hospital department under the auspices of the Medical Director. Referrals for specific treatment objectives are made by medical personnel directly to the music therapist. Such programs generally have a wide variety of components and serve multiple purposes. The primary purpose is to provide clinical music therapy services in accordance with established medical music therapy practices and approved hospital protocols.

Many hospitals also serve as an AMTA national training site for music therapy interns. Persons having completed their coursework for the bachelor's degree spend a minimum of 900 clinical hours under the supervision of a clinical music therapist. Additionally, some sites located in close proximity to a university offering a degree program may also provide training and supervision for music therapy majors in clinical practica. These students are completing 300 clinical hours while taking university coursework in the major. A few highly specialized medical music therapy programs also conduct research for development of innovative clinical practice.

Clinical Goals

Medical music therapy programs can occur in any medical service area including inpatient medical treatment, outpatient surgery and treatment, community education and wellness programs for prevention. The following goals come from the medical music therapy program at Tallahassee Memorial Hospital. Some were established by Jennifer Whipple, MT-BC, the first music therapist there, and others were developed by Darcy Walworth, MT-BC. They are indicative of the comprehensive scope of treatment possibilities in the medical environment.

Oncology Inpatient and Outpatient Units

- reduction or management of pain
- reduction or management of anxiety
- reduction of nausea during chemotherapy treatments
- counseling
- facilitation of effective communication with medical staff concerning treatment
- facilitation of desired communication with family and friends
- bereavement and counseling of family members

Pediatric Unit

- pain management or reduction
- enhancement of physical, occupational, and speech and language therapy goals
- stimulation and entertainment
- individual counseling with children and their families
- facilitation of effective communication for expressions of discomfort or distress
- bonding with medical staff to "humanize" the medical process.

Heart Institute Inpatient and Outpatient

- reduction of depression, anxiety and stress due to long-term hospitalization and lifestyle changes
- reduction or management of pain
- stimulation during long-term deprivation
- music for expressing joy and gratitude when a transplant occurs
- relaxation
- counseling

Neurology Inpatient and Outpatient

- enhancement of physical rehabilitation
- enhancement of speech and language therapy goals
- rehabilitation of short and long-term memory
- facilitating awareness of coma patients
- support groups for patients and families
- counseling
- stimulation during long-term hospitalization.

Extended Care/Long-Term Care and Geriatric Programs

- stimulation and entertainment
- anxiety reduction
- memory and cognitive stimulation for Alzheimer's patients
- enhancement of physical rehabilitation

Labor and Delivery

- reduction in length of labor
- increased relaxation during labor
- celebration of birth

Surgical Services

- anxiety reduction or management
- reduced need for anesthesia
- decreased time in recovery room
- pain reduction or management
- shortened hospital stay

Community Education Programs

- stress reduction or management
- pain reduction or management
- coping with lifestyle changes
- reduction of substance abuse

- controlling symptoms of debilitating diseases such as Alzheimer's, Parkinson's, Osteochondritis dissecans (OCD)
- support or counseling for families and caregivers of patients with debilitating diseases

In-Hospital Hospice Programs

- pain reduction
- anxiety reduction
- counseling
- management and control of life decisions during the dying process
- family communication and bereavement
- celebration of life

Newborn Intensive Care Goals

- pacification for growth and development
- enhancement of respiration and reduction of need for oxygen
- reinforcement of non-nutritive sucking
- parent training
- counseling for parents
- promotion of developmental skills such as awareness and tracking of auditory and visual stimuli, social reciprocity skills, and language development.

References

Aldridge, K. (1993). The use of music to relieve pre-operational anxiety in children attending day surgery. *The Australian Journal of Music Therapy*, 4, 19-35.

Ammon, K. (1968). The effects of music on children in respiratory distress. *American Nurses' Association Clinical Sessions*, 127-133.

Bailey, L. (1986). Music therapy in pain management. *Journal of Pain and Symptom Management*, 1(1), 25-28.

Brodsky, W. (1989). Music therapy as an intervention for children with cancer in isolation rooms. *Music Therapy*, 8, 17-34.

Burke, M., Walsh, J., Oehler, J., & Gingras, J. (1995). Music therapy following suctioning: Four case studies. *Neonatal Network*, 14(7), 41-49.

Caine, J. (1991). The effects of music on the selected stress behaviors, weight, caloric and formula intake, and length of hospital stay of premature and low birth weight neonates in a newborn intensive care unit. *Journal of Music Therapy*, 28(4), 180-192.

Caire, J., & Erickson, S. (1986). Reducing distress in pediatric patients undergoing cardiac catheterization. *Children's Health Care*, 14(3), 146-152.

Cassidy, J. W., & Ditty, K. M. (1998). Presentation of aural stimuli to newborns and premature infants: An audiological perspective. *Journal of Music Therapy*, 35(2), 70-87.

Cassidy, J. W., & Standley, J. M. (1995). The effect of music listening on physiological responses of premature infants in the NICU. *Journal of Music Therapy*, 32(4), 208-227.

Chapman, J. S. (1975). *The relation between auditory stimulation of short gestation infants and their gross motor limb activity*. Unpublished doctoral dissertation, New York University.

Chetta, H. D. (1981). The effect of music and desensitization on pre-operative anxiety in children. *Journal of Music Therapy*, 18, 74-87.

Clinton, P. K. (1984). *Music as a nursing intervention for children during painful procedures.* Unpublished master's thesis, The University of Iowa.

Cohen, A. (1984). *The development and implementation of a pediatric music therapy program in a short-term medical facility.* Unpublished master's thesis, New York University.

Coleman, J. M., Pratt, R. R., Stoddard, R. A., Gerstmann, D. R., & Abel, H. H. (1997). The effects of the male and female singing and speaking voices on selected physiological and behavioral measures of premature infants in the intensive care unit. *International Journal of Arts Medicine*, 5(2), 4-11.

Collins, S., & Kuck, K. (1991). Music therapy in the neonatal intensive care unit. *Neonatal Network*, 9(6), 23-26.

Corah, N., Gale, E., Pace, L., & Seyrek, S. (1981). Relaxation and musical programming as means of reducing psychological stress during dental procedures. *Journal of the American Dental Association*, 103, 232-234.

Davis, W., Gfeller, K., & Thaut, M. (1992). *An Introduction to music therapy theory and practice.* Dubuque, IA: Wm. C. Brown.

Fagen, T. (1982). Music therapy in the treatment of anxiety and fear in terminal pediatric patients. *Music Therapy*, 2, 13-23.

Farnsworth, P. (1958). *The social psychology of music.* New York: Holt, Rinehart, & Winston.

Flowers, A. L., McCain, A. P., & Hilker, K. A. (1999). *The effects of music listening on premature infants.* Paper presented at the Biennial Meeting, Society for Research in Child Development, April 15-18, Albuquerque, New Mexico.

Fowler-Kerry, S., & Lander, J. (1987). Management of injection pain in children. *Pain*, 30, 169-175.

Froelich, M. (1984). A comparison of the effect of music therapy and medical play therapy on the verbalization behavior of pediatric patients. *Journal of Music Therapy*, 21, 2-15.

Gettel, M. (1985). *The effect of music on anxiety in children undergoing cardiac catheterization.* Unpublished master's thesis, Hahnemann University.

Hanser, S. (1985). Music therapy and stress reduction research. *Journal of Music Therapy*, 22, 193-206.

Hoffman, J. (1980). *Management of essential hypertension through relaxation training with sound.* Unpublished master's thesis, University of Kansas.

Kamps, M. (1992). *The effects of singing on the respiratory abilities of cystic fibrosis patients.* Unpublished research paper, The Florida State University.

Katz, V. (1971). Auditory stimulation and developmental behavior of the premature infant. *Nursing Research*, 20, 196-201.

Lane, D. L. (1991). The effect of a single music therapy session on hospitalized children as measured by salivary Immunoglobulin A, speech pause time, and a patient opinion Likert scale. *Pediatric Research*, 29(4, Part 2), 11A.

Larson, K., & Ayllon, T. (1990). The effects of contingent music and differential reinforcement on infantile colic. *Behavior Research Therapy*, 28(2), 119-125.

Light, G., Love, D., Benson, D., & Morch, E. (1954). Music in surgery. *Current Researches in Anesthesia and Analgesia*, 33, 258-264.

Lindsay, K. (1981). The value of music for hospitalized infants. *Journal of the Association for the Care of Children in Hospitals*, 9(4), 104-107.

Lorch, C. A., Lorch, V., Diefendorf, A. O., & Earl, P. W. (1994). Effect of stimulative and sedative music on systolic blood pressure, heart rate, and respiratory rate in premature infants. *Journal of Music Therapy*, 31(2), 105-118.

Malloy, G. (1979). The relationship between maternal and musical auditory stimulation and the developmental behavior of premature infants. *Birth Defects: Original Article Series*, 15(7), 81-98.

Malone, A. B. (1996). The effects of live music on the distress of pediatric patients receiving intravenous starts, venipunctures, injections, and heel sticks. *Journal of Music Therapy*, 33(1), 19-33.

Marley, L. (1984). The use of music with hospitalized infants and toddlers: A descriptive study. *Journal of Music Therapy*, 21(3), 126-132.

McDonnell, L. (1984). Music therapy with trauma patients and their families on a pediatric service. *Music Therapy*, 4, 55-66.

Micci, N. (1984). The use of music therapy with pediatric patients undergoing cardiac catheterization. *The Arts in Psychotherapy*, 11, 261-266.

Miller, L. (1984). *Spontaneous music therapy sessions for hospitalized children.* Unpublished research paper, The Florida State University.

Moore, R., Gladstone, I., & Standley, J. (1994). *Effects of music, maternal voice, intrauterine sounds and white noise on the oxygen saturation levels of premature infants.* Unpublished paper presented at the National Conference, National Association for Music Therapy, Inc., November, Orlando, Florida.

Pfaff, V., Smith, K., & Gowan, D. (1989). The effects of music-assisted relaxation on the distress of pediatric cancer patients undergoing bone marrow aspirations. *Children's Health Care*, 18(4), 232-236.

Rasco, C. (1992). Using music therapy as distraction during lumbar punctures. *Journal of Pediatric Oncology Nursing*, 9(1), 33-34.

Robb, S. L., Nichols, R. J., Rutan, R. L., Bishop, B. L., & Parker, J. C. (1995). The effects of music assisted relaxation on preoperative anxiety. *Journal of Music Therapy*, 32(1), 2-21.

Robinson, D. (1962). Music therapy in a general hospital. *Bulletin of the National Association for Music Therapy*, 11(3), 13-18.

Rudenberg, M. T., & Royka, A. M. (1989). Promoting psychosocial adjustment in pediatric burn patients through music therapy and child life therapy. *Music Therapy Perspectives*, 7, 40-43.

Schneider, F. (1982). *Assessment and evaluation of audio-analgesic effects on the pain experience of acutely burned children during dressing changes.* Unpublished doctoral dissertation, University of Cincinnati.

Schwankovsky, L., & Guthrie, P. (1982). *Music therapy for handicapped children: Other health impaired.* NAMT Monograph Series. Washington, DC: National Association for Music Therapy.

Siegel, S. L. (1983). *The use of music as treatment in pain perception with post surgical patients in a pediatric hospital.* Unpublished master's thesis, The University of Miami.

Standley, J. (1991a). Long-term benefits of music intervention in the newborn intensive care unit: A pilot study. *Journal of the International Association of Music for the Handicapped,* 6(1), 12-23.

Standley, J. M. (2002a). *Music techniques in therapy, counseling, and special education.* St. Louis, MO: MMB, Inc., 2nd ed.

Standley, J. M. (1991b). The role of music in pacification/stimulation of premature infants with low birthweights. *Music Therapy Perspectives,* 9, 19-25.

Standley, J. M. (1998). The effect of music and multimodal stimulation on physiological and developmental responses of premature infants in neonatal intensive care. *Pediatric Nursing,* 24(6), 532-539.

Standley, J. M. (2000a). The effect of contingent music to increase non-nutritive sucking of premature infants. *Pediatric Nursing,* 26(5), 493-495, 498-499.

Standley, J. M. (2000b). Music research in medical/dental treatment: an update of a prior meta-analysis. In American Music Therapy Association (Ed.), *Effectiveness of music therapy procedures: Documentation of research and clinical practice* (3rd ed., pp. 1-60). Silver Spring, MD: American Music Therapy Association.

Standley, J. M. (2002b). A meta-analysis of the efficacy of music therapy for premature infants. *Journal of Pediatric Nursing,* 17(2), 107-113.

Standley, J. M. (2003). The effect of music-reinforced non-nutritive sucking on feeding rate of premature infants. *Journal of Pediatric Nursing.*

Standley, J. M., & Hanser, S. (1994, October). Music therapy research and applications in pediatric oncology treatment. *Journal of Pediatric Oncology Nursing.*

Standley, J. M., & Moore, R. S. (1995). Therapeutic effects of music and mother's voice on premature infants. *Pediatric Nursing,* 21(6), 509-512, 574.

Steinke, W. (1991). The use of music, relaxation, and imagery in the management of postsurgical pain for scoliosis. In C. D. Maranto (Ed.), *Applications of music in medicine* (pp. 141-162). Washington, DC: National Association for Music Therapy.

Taylor, D. (1981). Music in general hospital treatment from 1900 to 1950. *Journal of Music Therapy,* 18, 62-73.

Wagner, M. (1994). *Introductory musical acoustics.* Raleigh, NC: Contemporary Publishing.

Whipple, J. (2000). The effect of parent training in music and multimodal stimulation on parent-neonate interactions in the Neonatal Intensive Care Unit. *Journal of Music Therapy,* 37(4), 250-268.

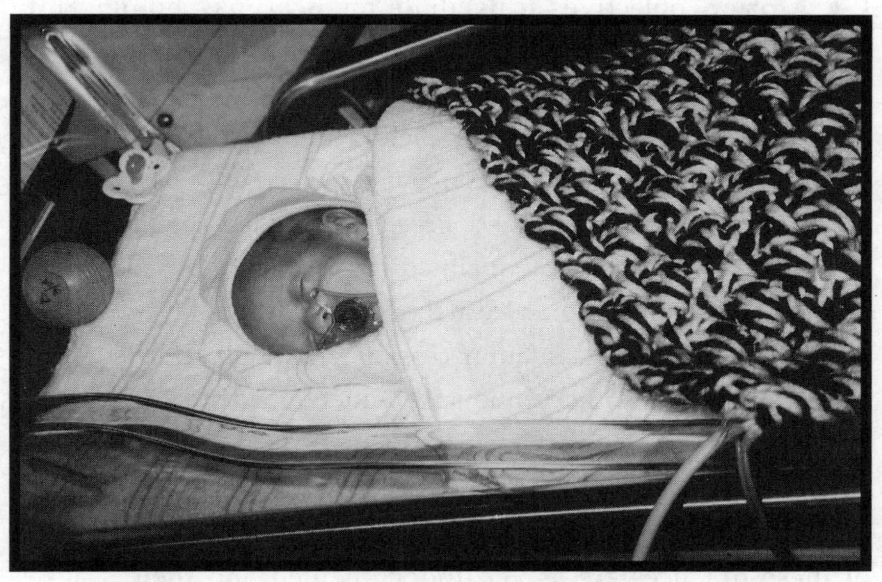

Libby has graduated to an open crib. She is ready for multimodal music therapy stimulation and encouragement of non-nutritive sucking.

3 | Music Therapy in the NICU

Music therapy is a research-based profession with specific a priori objectives to faciliate medical, psychological, or educational goals. Ongoing documentation of effectiveness for accountability is a standard element of clinical procedures derived from the research literature. For each procedure recommended in this chapter, the research in the area is reviewed and "best practice" clinical procedures synthesized. Practices included herein are those developed and utilized by qualified music therapists who require specialized training for practice in the NICU. The fragility and unique needs of the premature infant necessitate thorough knowledge and training prior to any intervention. Well-intentioned but unresearched practices have included harpists in the NICU, earth drums to simulate the sound of the mother's heart, classical music recordings, and piped-in music including that from radio stations. The effects of these practices are as yet undocumented and their usage is questionable at this time.

Specialized Training for NICU Music Therapy

Qualifications

The following people are qualified to complete specialized training in NICU music therapy: Board Certified Music Therapists preparing to provide NICU services; Qualified music therapy faculty at AMTA Approved Educational Programs with an established NICU liaison; and graduate and advanced music therapy majors in these programs. First, NICU Music Therapy trainees should review confidentiality and liability issues as mandated by the risk management division of the hospital in which they will provide services and acquire professional practice liability insurance. Then, specialized training can begin.

Training Curriculum

The curriculum for NICU music therapy training entails knowledge and understanding of:

- nursery protocols for clinical services, interdisciplinary team roles for assessment and treatment planning, and involvement of parents in treatment decisions;
- professional confidentiality regarding infants and families, particularly with regard to life-sustaining treatment or its cessation, paternity issues, socioeconomic factors, very young mothers making decisions for their infants, and lifestyles;
- nonjudgmental acceptance of infants' status and parent/staff decisions regarding treatment or its withholding;
- health issues, including importance of not coming to the nursery when exhibiting symptoms such as cold, runny nose, diarrhea, fever, fever blister, exposure to chicken pox;
- safety issues such as women not wearing artificial nails which can house and spread bacteria;
- universal precautions in the presence of bodily fluids, use of gloves, and avoidance of needles and disposal bins;
- scrubbing and glove requirements for diapering or stimulating infants as indicated by the medical staff;

- discrimination of permissive interactions such as diapering, holding and rocking infants, offering a pacifier versus non-permissive interactions such as feeding;
- requirements for students in training to be accompanied by a qualified music therapy faculty or staff member on all occasions in the NICU;
- the necessity for daily approval from the primary nursing caregiver to provide music therapy for an individual infant;
- music therapy techniques for premature infants;
- recognition of warning signs of infant distress and protocols for discontinuation of interaction;
- knowledge of medical conditions and treatments affecting premature infants' ability to participate in music therapy interventions.

Sound Levels in the NICU

Long-term implications of specific sound levels of music presentation are as yet unknown. The research and clinical literature on music listening and premature infants listening to music reports diverse dB sound levels measured on both Scales A and C and presentation modes including free field speakers, earphones, or ear cups. Neonatal audiologists recommend use of extreme caution with regard to the fragility of the developing infant's hearing ability and they consider all variables, loudness, duration, and presentation of auditory stimuli, to be of critical concern. All presentation modes seem to have pros and cons. Complete audiology information on the premature infant has been meticulously summarized by Cassidy and Ditty (1998) with resulting recommendations for sound presentation to premature infants provided according to specific variables (see Table 4).

Table 4. Considerations for Presentation of Stimuli

Considerations for Presentation of Stimuli

FREE FIELD (Open Incubators and Radient Warmers)		**EAR CUPS**	
Positive	**Things to Consider**	**Positive**	**Things to Consider**
Diffusion of sound helps if dB too loud	Decibel levels must be measured at ear, not at source	Much more control over decibel level	Must purchase expensive audiological equipment to use
Easy	Will not completely mask ambient noise	Attenuates ambient noise, allowing for minimum volume	Ear cups are sterile, disposable, and expensive
Inexpensive	Other infants in nursery may hear music	Guarantees binaural presentation of stimulus	Ear cups are not readily available—must be ordered
	Place single speaker at midline of body—close to ears is best	No effect on other infants in nursery Baby can lay on side or back without collapsing ear canal	Stimulation is tactile as well as auditory Decibel measurements should be made with a coupler
FREE FIELD (Closed Incubator)		**PHONOPAD EARPHONES**	
Positive	**Things to Consider**	**Positive**	**Things to Consider**
May attenuate outside sounds	Decibel levels must be measured for each child at ear, not at source	Much more control over decibel level Attenuates ambient noise, allowing for minimum volume	Equipment must be sterilized There is variation in decibel levels from one headset to another
Will not affect other babies	Size of space inside incubator with baby will change for each child, affects dB	Guarantees binaural presentation of stimulus when carefully placed	Decibel measurements should be made with a coupler
Easy	Place single speaker at midline of body—close to ears is best	No effect on other infants in nursery	Decibel level is critical because the ear canal is blocked leaving very small resonating chamber
Inexpensive	Sound level should be set softer than in open incubator	Relatively inexpensive equipment	Phonopads can be put inside fold of infant cap to hold in place.
EAR MUFFS, HEADPHONES		**SOMATRON**	
Positive	**Things to Consider**	**Positive**	**Things to Consider**
Much more control over decibel level	Equipment must be sterilized	Bed could be placed away from noise in NICU	Expensive equipment
Attenuates ambient noise, allowing for minimum volume	There is variation in decibel levels from one headset to another	More comfortable for infant than cumbersome headphones	Stimulation would be multimodal*
Guarantees binaural presentation of stimulus	Decibel measurements should be made with a coupler	No effect on other infants in nursery	Decibel levels reaching eardrum would be difficult to measure
No effect on other infants in nursery	Baby must be on back for binaural presentation	**LIVE-SINGING**	
Fairly inexpensive and readily available	Stimulation is tactile as well as auditory	**Positive**	**Things to Consider**
		No equipment necessary so less concern with decibel level	Should there be multimodal stimulation ?
		Most natural form of infant musical stimulation	Hold baby in correct position for binaural listening
		Allows parents to bond with infant	Singer use appropriately soft and calm singing voice

*Assure that child is mature enough for multimodal stimulation   Table reprinted with permission from Cassidy & Ditty (1998), pp. 80-81.

It is noted that the American Academy of Pediatrics Committee on Environmental Health (1997) has recommended that environmental noise levels within the NICU be kept below 55 dB on Scale A due to concerns about long-term exposure to aversive auditory stimuli. Music is acoustically different from noise. Recommended dB levels for optional sound provision and for differentiation of music intended to pacify vs. stimulate are still evolving. All music therapy procedures in this book will reference existing literature for recommended sound levels.

Presentation Modes for Auditory Stimuli

Music stimuli are usually presented individually for maximum therapeutic benefit in the NICU. Obviously, presentation mode needs to be carefully considered with premature infants and all modes have some inherent drawbacks. Ear cups attached to audiological insert phones have been used to present the music stimulus to infants (Cassidy & Standley, 1995). With this equipment, it is assured that each infant is presented the stimulus at the same carefully controlled decibel level and that the decibel level is comfortable for the infant. The use of ear cups expand the resonating chamber to include the ear canal and the ear cup itself. Using ear cups, decibel levels can be set without regard to the size of ear canals. Unfortunately, audiological insert phones are quite expensive (approximately $750) as are the ear cups ($40/pair, one sterile pair/infant).

Music has also been presented via phonopad earphones positioned over each ear in the fold of the infant's knitted cap (Standley & Moore, 1995). With this mode of presentation, the ear canal is blocked off thereby creating a very small resonating chamber. Results from research in audiology indicate that an average of 7-15 dB correction is necessary for more accurate approximations of real-ear measurements of newborns and infants due to differences in ear canal volume (Stelmachowicz, 2000). This means that an adult ear with a relatively large ear canal (i.e., resonating chamber) would hear an 80 dB sound as 80 dB, whereas a newborn would hear that same tone as anywhere from 87 to 95 dB, or 7 to 15 dB louder. Premature infants' ear canals are even smaller and therefore the difference is probably greater, but their hearing thresholds are also higher due to neurological immaturity. The 65 to 70 dB volume settings of the previous study and other music studies with premature infants (Caine, 1992; Collins & Kuck, 1991) may have been perceived as much louder. Measurement of dependent variables did not demonstrate negative effects of this volume level. It should be noted that phonopad earphones are difficult to place in exactly the same position for all infants. Since ear canal sizes vary by infant, all calculations of appropriate dB levels are very difficult (Cassidy & Ditty, 1998).

A third alternative for presentation mode is a tape recorder with binaural speakers placed on both sides of the infant's head. Unfortunately, such placement of speakers in the incubator may not mask environmental noise as effectively as ear couplers or earphones.

It is apparent that presentation modes vary widely depending upon multiple variables. Careful consideration should be given to this issue and mode dictated by the infant's environment, gestational age, and purpose of music presentation.

NICU Music Therapy (MT) Techniques

Music Effects on NICU Ambient Sound Levels

Noise in the NICU results in detrimental infant responses: reduced oxygen saturation levels, rise in heart and respiratory rate, and change in behavioral state from quiet to fussy crying (Zahr & Balian, 1995). Infants in single versus double-walled incubators have greater physiological decreases to sound (Yeh, Voora, & Lilien, 1980).

The effect of free field music on sound levels were studied in a NICU which was a large, open area crowded with people and busy with activity. The census during the period of the study averaged 10-12 infants. At all times during the sound level measurements there were three or four nursing personnel in the room, three music therapists, and the observer recording sound levels. Frequently, there were two or more parents in the room. Additionally, other staff came in periodically to conduct medical tests or interventions. Activities during these measurements included singing and massaging infants, parental kangaroo parent care, bathing and dressing, feeding, medical procedures, answering parents inquiries via telephone, and staff organization and communication.

The music equipment added to the space consisted of a CD player connected to a Paradox wireless audio system with a remote transmitter and two wireless speakers placed on shelves approximately 18" from the ceiling. The speakers were positioned at each end of the unit about 1/4 of the length of the room and diagonally facing the center of the room. The controls were set on the CD and on each speaker such that the music volume throughout the room varied from 61-62 dB (Scale C measured outside each isolette at about infant head level using a digital sound level meter.)

Music content was limited to 13 commercial CDs which were selected, numbered, and placed on the unit. All selections were made by the experimenter based on volume range, homogeneous sound, and soothing qualities. Included were lullaby music by male and female vocalists, instrumental lullaby music, instrumental classical music, and instrumental music composed especially for healthcare environments. Nursing personnel were free to select from among the provided CDs and were asked to log daily the identifying number and duration of each CD played. At the end of the experiment, the daily logs were analyzed for music preference, daily duration of music, and frequency/selection. Table 5 shows selections by order of playing preference. Overall, duration analysis showed a daily 24-hour mean of 2.6 hours of music for the length of the experiment.

Table 5. Nurses' Music Preference by Percent Play Time

% Play Time	Artist	Album Title	Year	Company
18	Instrumental	*Music for Dreaming*	1994	Sony Music Entertainment
14	Nicolette Larson	*Sleep, Baby, Sleep*	1994	Sony Music Entertainment
14	Olivia Newton-John	*Warm and Tender*	1989	Geffen Records, Inc.
12	Instrumental	*Build Your Baby's Brain* (free CD to babies in GA)	1998	Sony Music Entertainment
8	Instrumental	*HeartSong*	1997	Healing HealthCare Systems, Inc.
7	Instrumental	*Baby Sleep*	1996	Warner Music
7	Various Artists	*Disney Babies Lullaby*	1988	Walt Disney Records
7	Joanie Bartels	*Lullaby Magic*		Discovery Music
4	Connie Kaldo & Carmen Campagne	*Lullaby Berceuse*	1996	Coyote Prod., Music for Little People
4	Priscilla Herdman	*Star Dreamer*	1988	Alcazam
2	Various Artists	*A Child's Celebration of Lullaby*	1997	Music for Little People
2	Various Artists	*Daddies Sing Good Night*	1994	Sugar Hill Records
1	Mickey Dolenz	*Mickey Dolenz Puts You to Sleep*	1991	Rhino Records

NICU sound levels were measured weekly or bi-weekly for a total of 10 measures in 7 weeks in the Intermediate NICU before, during, and after music onset. Decibel levels were recorded at the same spot in the center of the room each minute for 10 minutes prior to music, 30 minutes during music, and for 10 minutes following music cessation. Simultaneously recorded each minute were yes/no determinations of whether any monitor alarms were sounding, whether talking was occurring, whether anyone was singing with the music, and whether any infants were crying. Reliability on the observation form between independent observers was .91.

The 10 average dB levels for pre, during, and post music time periods were calculated and subjected to one-way analysis of variance. Results were not statistically significant. Analysis of the incidence of monitor alarms, talking, singing, and crying showed that all decreased slightly during music (Figure 4). Primarily, music functioned to decrease talking in the NICU. Mean dB levels for the 1st and 7th weeks were graphed to ascertain effects across time. Figure 5 shows that decibel levels decreased during music periods across the first and last weeks.

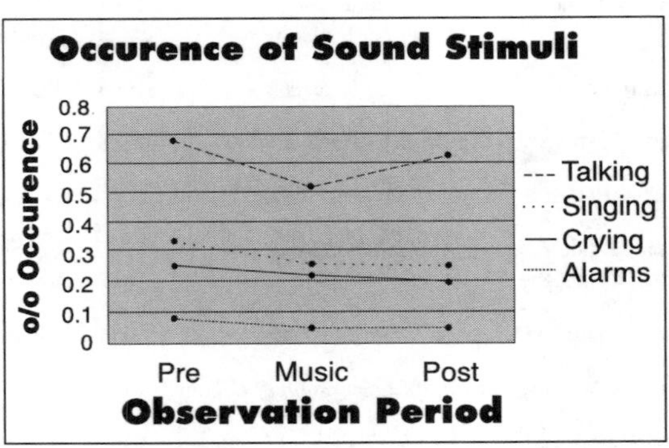

Figure 4. Occurrence of Sound Stimuli

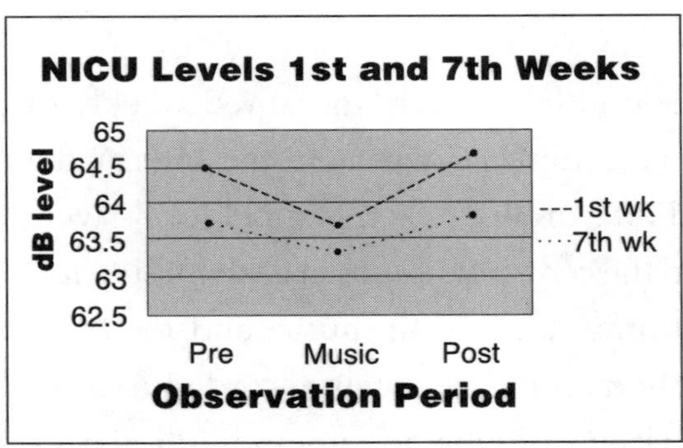

Figure 5. NICU dB Levels 1st and 7th Weeks

Research on Individually Provided Periods of Sustained Music

Respiratory functions are a critical problem for the very premature infant. Respiratory regularity and oxygen saturation levels are directly affected by the infant's behavioral state and degree of pain (Gordin, 1990). Loud noises disturb sleep, generate startle responses, elicit crying, and decrease oxygen saturation levels. It has been noted that staff in medical rounds approaching the incubator cause babies to exhibit more bradycardic and apneic episodes (Gorski, Davison, & Brazelton, 1979).

Music research has shown excellent benefits for premature infants' respiration. In fact, all prolonged auditory stimuli with a regular rhythm seem to pacify normal infants and regulate respiration. Salk made claims for the superiority of heartbeat in this capacity, but subsequent research has shown that it is the regularity of sound, not the heartbeat itself, that pacifies (Detterman, 1978). More than a decade ago, neonatology researchers became intrigued with the potential of music applications to mask aversive environmental auditory stimuli and to reduce the high risk for complications or failure to thrive in these infants (Leonard, 1993; Oehler, 1993; Standley, 1991). Indeed, an early study by Chapman (1979) found that infants receiving music combined with movement in the isolette had a 16% reduced length of hospitalization. A subsequent study by Caine (1992) found that music played 1.5 hours/ day throughout the NICU stay significantly reduced the total length of hospitalization for premature infants. Collins and Kuck (1991) observed 17 agitated premature infants under music and silence conditions. Oxygen saturation levels were significantly increased by this one 10-minute trial of auditory stimulation.

Psychological research with term infants revealed a preference for the mother's voice above all other auditory stimuli on the first day of life (DeCasper & Fifer, 1980). Auditory preference may be an important factor in regulating respiratory responses of premature infants and it was theorized that the mother's voice might be more effective than music in pacification. The mother's voice added to the NICU environment might also facilitate infant bonding. This theory was tested by Standley and Moore (1995). Subjects were 20 premature infants receiving oxygen. Two groups were matched with regard to sex, age, and weight with 10 subjects listening to music and 10 listening to a recording of their mother's voice. Dependent variables were oxygen saturation levels and occurrences of Oximeter alarms recorded at 2-minute intervals during auditory (20 minutes) and pre/post silence conditions (10 minutes each) across three days. Commercially recorded lullabies sung by female vocalists versus a recording of each infant's mother talking to her child were the independent variable. Auditory stimuli were provided via tape recorders and Sony phonopad earphones.

On Day 1, the music stabilized and significantly increased oxygen saturation levels, especially during the second 10-minute period ($t=2.40$, $df=8$, $p<.05$). On Days 2 and 3, there were no significant differences between groups during auditory stimulation.

Activation of an Oximeter alarm denoted a drop in oxygen saturation levels below 87%, requiring an immediate medical response. Mean alarm activations by listening interval across the three days were calculated for each subject and groups compared. The music group showed a significantly decreased rate of alarms ($t=2.675$, $df=18$, $p<.05$). Music functioned to stabilize respiration rate of the premature infants.

A study by Cassidy and Standley (1995) observed physiological responses of severely premature infants under music listening conditions as compared to normal environmental sounds. Every minute for 36 minutes during three consecutive days data were collected on oxygen saturation levels, heart rate, and respiratory rate.

Also noted from the medical charts were instances of apnea and bradycardia for the 24 hours preceding and following data collection. Music immediately and positively affected oxygen saturation levels, heart rate, and respiration rate on Day 1. Acclimation to the music stimuli resulted in more minimal effects on these physiological responses on Days 2 and 3. These findings are consistent with prior research in this area. This study demonstrated no negative effects on apnea/bradycardia. It also clarifies several issues for clinical application of music in the NICU.

Coleman, Pratt, Stoddard, Gerstmann, and Abel (1999) found that music lowered heart rate, increased oxygen saturation, reduced distress behaviors, and decreased time in hospital and that infants responded equally to male and female voices. It was also determined that music provided closer to birth date of the infants was more effective. Moore, Gladstone, and Standley (1994) tested music versus silence, mother's voice reading poetry, uterine noise, and white noise on 30-32 AGA week infants. All auditory stimuli were better than silence and did not differentially affect oxygen saturation levels. It was concluded that infants were too young to discriminate among auditory stimuli, but that sound was preferable to silence. Flowers, McCain, and Hilker (1999) compared music with womb sounds to radio music and normal NICU environmental sounds. Again, the lullabies with womb sounds had the greatest effects on physiological measures and behavioral state.

These data demonstrate that there is no evidence to contraindicate music listening in the first weeks of life for even very fragile premature babies (1 lb, 5 oz. to 3 lbs). Additionally, favorable long-term benefits of music are noticeable. Under peaceful sleeping conditions, neonates exhibit higher and more stable oxygen saturation levels, slower respiratory rates, and more stable heart rates (although the actual heart rate is dependent on numerous variables including gender and medication). To the extent that these trends are notable, music appears to relax and comfort these usually irritable infants. As in the Standley and Moore study (1995), it seems that music has its greatest effect on the first day of presentation. After the novelty has worn off, effects appear less noticeable as perhaps these infants are acclimating to their normally noisy environment by "turning off" sound perception. As a rule, all of these infants are placed on minimal stimulation during the early weeks of life; however, environmental auditory stimulation is much more difficult to control in an intensive care unit than other sensory stimuli. Therefore, one might expect that presentation of music would, at the very least, be no more stimulating than their normal environment. At best, it would be soothing, be predictable, and would mask other environmental sounds.

MT Intervention I:
Sustained Music, Live or Recorded, Provided Individually

Goals: Facilitation of growth, development, and learning; increased respiration capabilities; and reduction of stress.

Objectives and Documentation

- To increase oxygen saturation while reducing oxygen levels. *Measure oxygen saturation levels at regular intervals throughout music provision, record number of alarms indicating desaturation below 87%, record level of oxygen provision at start of music and all adjustments during music provision.*
- To regulate respiration following extubation. *Measure respiration rate at regular intervals throughout music provision, record number of apnea/bradycardia episodes, measure length of time from extubation to re-intubation, if necessary.*
- To increase opportunities for auditory processing, neurological growth, and development. *Measure head circumference weekly, record days to discharge from hospital, assess skills at discharge on the Brazelton Neonatal Behavioral Scale.*
- To provide auditory respite from noise-induced stress. *Observe and record infant state at regular intervals throughout music provision. Measure ambient noise level in NICU before, during, and after music provision.*
- To increase opportunity for language input. *Document language content of auditory stimuli presented.*

Infant Criteria

- Infant should be at least 28 weeks GA. Auditory brainstem responses are obtained as early as 26 weeks gestation (Cox, Martin, Carlo, & Hack, 1993) with consistent auditory responses obtained at 28 weeks. Therefore, it is assumed that newborns of greater than 28 weeks gestation might benefit from early auditory stimulation.

- Medical status should be stable. Note that music will have different impact for males vs. females due to gender differences in hearing acuity: infant male hearing is less developed than that of females.

Daily Nursing Approval

This procedure will require daily approval of the nurse providing care to the individual infant. He/she must verify that the infant could benefit from sound stimulation before music begins. Often the infant has endured medical procedures, is ill, is demonstrating symptoms of overstimulation, or is generally in need of the greatest amount of rest possible. The infant's nurse is the best authority to decide if it is appropriate to begin this procedure.

Selection of Auditory Stimuli

- Use music, not white noise, heart beats, or nature sounds.
- Use a variety of selections for developing auditory processing skills, not the same thing endlessly repeated which reduces learning and increases fatigue.
- Use the human voice for development of language.
- Use the voice preference of term infants: the mother, a female or other children.
- Use directed language when possible. Directed language is live, not recorded, and is interactive with an individual infant. It has language and social reciprocity (causal responses to the infant's responses). If the infant vocalizes, the person responds; if the infant startles, the person reduces the volume, speed, or emphasis of the sound, etc. Directed language may be sung.
- Changing auditory stimuli are alerting, therefore the music should be soothing, constant, stable, and relatively unchanging. Music should be as simple, non-alerting as possible in initial presentations or for very premature infants to facilitate habituation which equates with neurological maturation. Non-alerting music contains these elements:
    - voice unaccompanied or with a single accompanying instrument;
    - light rhythmic emphasis, constant rhythm;
    - constant volume;
    - melodies in the higher vocal ranges which infants hear best;
    - female vocalists (or child vocalists since term infants learn quickly from other children).
- Lullabies of all cultures meet the above criteria and promote language development due to an emphasis on vowels, rising/falling phrases, and the recognition of soothing sounds.

Music Volume

Use a volume level in the low 70s dB range on the C scale (never >75-80 dB). Care must be taken to set the loudness level individually to meet the readiness level for each infant, the logistics of their care environment, and to assure that nearby infants are not disturbed. Place speakers on each side of the infant's head so that sound stimuli are received binaurally.

Music Duration

The maximum time/day for sustained music is 1.5 hours, alternated ½ hour on and ½ hour off. Some babies may not be ready for this extended length of sound stimulation and the nurse may advise a shorter period. The impact of longer periods of music provision have not been researched.

Parent and Family Provision of Music. Parents may wish to provide their child with a small tape recorder with commercially recorded music approved by the NICU Music Therapist. Preferred music would be lullabies that maintain a constant accompaniment and tempo. A list of pre-approved lullaby tapes can be provided for the convenience of the parents and should reflect the cultural diversity of the many parents served in the NICU. A consultation with the Music Therapist should be available to assist parents in purchasing tape or CD players and recordings.

Parents may also wish to place recordings made especially for their baby. The mother's voice would be the most important for the baby to recognize and bond with. On this recording, the mother might read to the baby, talk to the baby, or sing lullabies. Research shows that the mother's voice is very important to the infant's recognition and that lullabies promote language development in infants. The most important thing is that the voice is steady, constant, and soothing with no abrupt starts, stops, or changes. Again, a consultation with the Music Therapist can assist the parents with plans for making such a tape.

Placement of musical toys and mobiles are contraindicated in the NICU due to the highly repetitive nature of the sole music selection usually available on these toys, the inability to adjust sound levels, and the lack of research on their use. If a parent has a special reason for wishing to use such a toy, a consultation with the Music Therapist would be indicated.

Parents, especially mothers, are encouraged during their visits to sing or speak to their babies to help them bond and learn to recognize the parent's voice. Again, this speaking should be in a quiet, sing/song or lullaby format with no abrupt changes so that infant stress is reduced. No approval is needed for this procedure unless the nurse detects signs of overstimulation and recommends that the parent discontinue the sound stimuli. A consultation with the Music Therapist should be available to provide training for this procedure and to teach detection of the early signs of overstimulation so that the parent would know when to stop the procedure.

Recommended Commercial Music Selections. There is no research to show that any particular piece or type of music is best for premature infants. However, we do know certain results about how infants are pacified by music and have identified characteristics of music for this purpose in the above treatment procedures. Commercial lullaby recordings were screened for these characteristics and are listed in Table 6. For variety, some recordings with male vocalists and some purely instrumental recordings which meet the majority of these criteria have been included.

Table 6. Commercial Recordings for Pacification

No.	Artist	Album	Year	Company
1	Nicolette Larson	*Sleep, Baby, Sleep*	1994	Sony Music Entertainment, Inc.
2	Joanie Bartels	*Lullaby Magic*	unknown	Discovery Music
3	Various artists	*Daddies Sing Good Night*	1994	Sugar Hill Records
4	Priscilla Herdman	*Star Dreamer*	1988	Alcazam
5	Connie Kaldor & Carmen Campagne	*Lullaby Berceuse*	1988, 1996	Coyote Productions Music for Little People
6	Various artists	*A Child's Celebration of Lullaby*	1997	Music for Little People
7	Olivia Newton-John	*Warm and Tender*	1989	Geffen Records, Inc.
8	Various artists	*Disney Babies Lullaby*	1988	Walt Disney Records
9	Instrumental	*Music for Dreaming*	1995	C.A. Ross
10	Mickey Dolenz	*Mickey Dolenz Puts You to Sleep*	1991	Rhino Records
11	Instrumental	*Baby Sleep*	1996	Warner Music
12	Instrumental	*HeartSong*	1997	Healing HealthCare Systems, Inc.

Research on Music and Non-Nutritive Sucking (NNS)

The newborn's ability to suck is critical for both survival and neurological development. The first rhythmic behavior in which the infant engages, sucking is theorized to contribute to neurological development by facilitating internally regulated rhythms (Goff, 1985). While non-nutritive sucking (NNS) is a reflex which appears with physiologic maturation, its effectiveness can be altered by learning experiences (Anderson & Vidyasagar, 1979; Bernbaum, Pereira, Watkins, & Peckham, 1983). Sucking behavior appears during the third trimester of fetal development. Unfortunately, NICU treatment constraints may inhibit NNS opportunity while very premature infants are completing their third trimester.

It is reassuring to note that NNS opportunities given in the NICU, enhance development of the premature infant. Pacifier use increases infant oxygenation (Burroughs, Asonye, Anderson-Shanklin, & Vidyasagar,1973). The coordinated suck-swallow-breathe response is a precursor to nutritive sucking ability and nipple feeding. Pacifiers offered during gavage feeding at this stage of development increase infants' daily weight gain (Field et al., 1982). It is theorized that NNS activates the vagal nerve which excites the release of gastrointestinal hormones, specifically gastrin and cholecystokinin. These hormones stimulate gastro-intestinal motoric and secretory activity, growth of the intestinal tract, release of glucose-induced insulin and enhancement of the infant's energy economy (Dieter & Emory, 1997). Thus, NNS promotes growth and development.

Music is effective reinforcement for learning in all ages of individuals and for diverse goals within educational, home, and health settings (Standley, 1996). DeCasper and Carstens (1981) demonstrated the effects of music reinforcement on sucking behavior of 2-day-old term infants. Research in contingent cause/effect learning of premature infants is sparse. Only one prior music study of this type has been identified. Schunk (1993) conducted a pilot study to determine whether background music played contingently during feeding could enhance weight gain of premature infants. The study had a very small sample size and results were inconclusive; however, positive changes in infant behavior were observed during music. She recommended further research, particularly with regard to individual feedback for ineffective sucking rates.

Standley (2000) conducted a study to determine whether pacifier activated lullaby music would reinforce NNS rates of premature infants who were evaluated as poor feeders in need of occupational therapist assistance. A secondary issue was whether premature infants would develop discrimination of on/off music stimuli.

The PAL (pacifier-activated-lullaby) device for this study consisting of a Minimam Newborn Orthodontic Pacifier by Ross Laboratories, #50486, was adapted so that a suck of predetermined strength activated an electrical signal to a cassette tape player. Pressure sensitivity and length of music activation could be controlled for each suck. Sensitivity was set at minimal pressure and music duration at 10 seconds with duration reset with each suck. Each music activation also activated red lights on the control box designating sucking frequency and duration. The duration indicator was used for data collection.

The study utilized subjects as their own control in a design of ABAB across 14 minutes. A silence condition for the first 2 minutes of baseline was followed by 5 minutes of contingent music, followed by another 2-minute period of silence and another 5 minutes of contingent music. The pacifier remained in the infants' mouths across the entire 14 minutes with only the availability of the music added or deleted according to condition.

The dependent variable was sucking duration/5-second interval recorded by two trained observers with 96% reliability. Trials occurred between 4-5 p.m. in the interval of at least 1 hour past the last feeding and at least 1 hour prior to the next feeding. The pacifier was carefully placed in the infant's mouth and held there with light pressure but with no further manipulation which might have activated sucking. Due to the fragility of these infants, it was planned to cease the trial if any infant distress symptoms occurred (Rauh, Nurcombe, Achenbach, & Howell, 1987). However, no instances of overstimulation were observed during this study.

The music tape included a selection of commercially recorded lullabies sung by female vocalists played free field (without earphones) at 65-70 dB measured at the tape recorder placed at the feet or to the lower side of the infant.

The mean number of 5-second intervals/minute in which the duration indicator was lit constituted the sucking rate for each child. Multivariate repeated measures analyses for experimental condition and gender were significant for condition only (see Table 7). The first silence condition was significant from all other conditions, and other relationships were not significant.

Table 7. Mean Sucking Rate/Minute for Each Condition

	Conditions			
	Silence 1	Music 1	Silence 2	Music 2
Mean Sucking Rates	3.00	7.28	5.42	7.60

Figure 6 shows a clear learning curve with sucking rates consistently increasing across time during the first contingent music interval then dropping substantially during the second baseline condition. Sucking rates were highest overall in the first minute of the second contingent music condition. It is also interesting to note that sucking rates during music were 2.43 times as great as those during silence. It is obvious that infant learning and discrimination of music occurred. The final music condition shows a steady decline in sucking rate attributed to fatigue or to the infant lulling him/herself to sleep prior to the end of the trial.

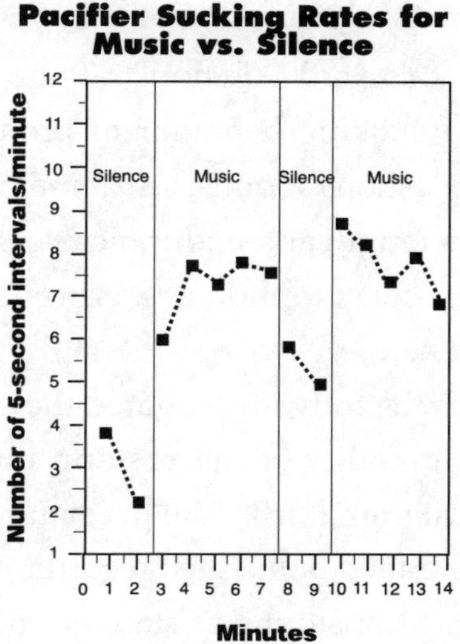

Graph reprinted by permission of Pediatric Nursing (Standley, 2000).
Figure 6. Pacifier Sucking Rates for Music vs. Silence

The sucking rate for sufficient endurance during feeding is unknown for premature infants. However, research has shown that the combined nutritive/non-nutritive sucking rate of newborn term infants (40 weeks gestation) across a 15-minute feeding interval is 65% (Rybski, Almli, Gisel, Powers, & Maurer, 1984). This rate is only slightly more than the 63% rate of 37.7 seconds per minute achieved in this study by premature infants referred for poor sucking responses and a need for occupational therapy. The music reinforcement increased premature non-nutritive sucking rates to combined nutritive/non-nutritive levels of term infants. These data provide a standard for developmental goals of premature infants.

It was observed during the study that the infants adapted to the music cutting on and off and showed no startle responses to these events. None of the subjects were observed to exhibit signs of overstimulation during or after the experimental trials. The contingent music intervention increased NNS with no negative side effects noted.

The results of this study demonstrate a viable intervention to "teach" prolonged sucking behavior to premature infants in the NICU, but many questions about its use remain. The optimal sucking time for building strength and endurance versus negative effects of fatigue and energy consumption at a critical time for weight gain requires delineation.

A second research study investigated the effect of PAL usage on subsequent feeding ability of the preterm infant (Standley, 2003). Due to neurological immaturity, the premature infant has impaired behavioral state organization. Cues regarding behavioral state are not easily read and transitions in state are not smooth. When the infant is immature, it is often poorly organized for feeding. Attempts at feeding result in heart rate increases and respiratory interruptions leading to apneic episodes. Sucking responses may be weak or uncoordinated. Thus, nutritive sucking in premature infants frequently reduces oxygen saturation, expends energy, and causes weight loss (Hill, 1992).

Prior to 34 weeks AGA, gavage feeding by oral-gastric or naso-gastric tube is necessary, but stressful, for the premature infant. The infants find the sensation of formula filling their stomach unpleasant and often resist by tensing the stomach muscles. This pushes the formula back up the tube and prolongs the feeding interval. Gavage feeding is beneficially paired with NNS and promotes infant development in a variety of ways. It lowers heart rate (McCain, 1995; Woodson & Hamilton, 1988), increases oxygenation (Burroughs et al., 1978), and increases weight gain of the infant even when nutritional intake is controlled (Field et al., 1982; Kanarek & Shulman,

1992). The lower activity levels facilitated by pacifier sucking result in energy conservation and subsequent weight gain. Non-nutritive sucking increases duration of inactive alert state and faster return to, and increased length of, quiet sleep (DiPietro, Cusson, Caughy, & Fox, 1994; Gill, Behnke, Conlon, McNeely, & Anderson, 1988; Goff, 1986; McCain, 1992, 1995). A meta-analysis on the clinical outcomes of NNS paired with gavage feeding found that it decreased length of hospitalization by an average of 6.3 days and allowed premature infants to begin bottle feeding an average of 2.9 days sooner (Schwartz, Moody, Yarndi, & Anderson, 1987).

The development of sucking ability for feeding is indicative of cognitive growth (Medoff-Cooper & Gennaro, 1996). Indeed, it correlates with neurological maturity not gestational age or birth weight (McCain, 1992). Medical procedures such as intubation can delay the development of a coordinated sucking pattern in premature infants. Transition from gavage to nipple feeding is often difficult for the premature infant and sometimes long-term problems develop such as nipple aversion or aversion to oral feeding (Palmer, 1993). Palmer's (1993) assessment of premature infants consistently found an immature pattern of sucking consisting of 3-5 sucks in a burst followed by a pause to breathe. More mature, term infants sucked 10-30 times in a prolonged burst and alternated breathing with sucking. Mature nutritive sucking coordination would seem to be a highly important goal for premature infants for a variety of health, growth, and developmental reasons.

Oral feeding skill can be assisted through NNS. Pacifiers given 10 minutes prior to nipple feeding increase the inactive awake state of the infant and decrease the total length of time for ingestion of nutrition (McCain, 1995). Due to adverse physiological reactions to prolonged feeding, the standard of care for premature infants usually limits a nipple feeding opportunity to 30 minutes with the remaining nutrition given by gavage (Gardner, Garland, Merenstein, & Lubchenco, 1997). Strengthening the suck and increasing the rate of nutritional intake is frequently a primary goal to reduce the length of a nipple feeding episode.

This study used the PAL to reinforce NNS of premature infants deemed poor feeders by NICU personnel and evaluated improvement in nipple feeding rate (Standley, 2003). Participants were 32 premature infants randomly divided between experimental and control groups. Multivariate analysis of variance showed no significant difference between the groups with regard to gestational age at birth, birth weight, AGA at time of study, weight at time of study, or age at time of study. Each infant had failed to make the transition to bottle feeding and was being given primarily gavage feedings with minimal opportunities each day for nipple feeding. Specific criteria for participation in the study were: ineffective nutritive sucking, age of approximately 34 weeks AGA, and ability to tolerate two simultaneous types of stimulation (pacifier and auditory stimulation).

The experimental group received one 15-20 minute trial with the PAL between 4-5 p.m., approximately 30-60 minutes prior to the late afternoon opportunity for nipple feeding. The control group received no PAL training. Data were recorded by the researcher from the nurses' notes who were blind to the purpose of the study and to infants' status in the study. Data included the nutritional amount ingested and length of feeding time for the nipple feeding opportunity in the morning and again in the evening for each infant on the selected day, either the date of PAL intervention or a randomly selected day during the week after referral for control infants. Volume ingested was divided by minutes of feeding to obtain individual nipple feeding rates.

Again, in this study the music consisted of a selection of commercially recorded lullabies sung by female vocalists played free field. The sound volume was approximately 65 dB(C)/58 dB(A) measured at the tape player.

A *t* test comparison was made between groups for morning feeding rates prior to PAL intervention. There was no significant difference between groups (t=-.259, df=30, α>.05). The *t* test comparison between groups for the late afternoon feeding rate (post PAL intervention) was significantly different (t=2.532, df=30, α<.05). Table 8 shows group means for these two intervals and demonstrates that the experimental infants increased feeding rates in the same afternoon following PAL presentation, a significant increase from the morning rate (t=2.875, df=15, α<.05). The control group, however, slightly decreased sucking rates in the afternoon (t=-2.116, df=15, α>.05). This was a nonsignificant decrease.

Table 8. Mean Feeding Rates by Group

	Pre Feeding Rate	Post Feeding Rate*
Experimental Group (n=16)	2.21 cc/min.	2.97 cc/min.
Control Group (n=16)	2.34 cc/min.	1.86 cc/min.

*Significant difference between groups, α<.05

One treatment for poor feeding skill in a premature infant of 36 or more weeks adjusted gestational age is referral to an Occupational Therapist who often uses a variety of physical manipulations to assist the infant in feeding. Palmer (1993) says this is contraindicated and the preferred methodology for assistance would be teaching the infant to pace his/her sucking pattern. The PAL's adjustable rate of music reinforcement provides just such pacing feedback. It is interesting to note that in the experimental opportunity, the infants appear to have practiced a skill that transferred to a new situation later in the day. In this NBICU the nurses often observe that some infants having difficulty making the transition to enteral feeding from gavage feeding over an extended period suddenly, one day, seem to "get it" as though a light bulb had come on. These infants then seem to have the skill for all future feedings. The PAL helped all of the experimental infants learn or "get it" in one trial. Music-reinforced NNS is an effective intervention for a very important developmental milestone.

MT Intervention II:
Music to Reinforce NNS Using the PAL[1]

Goals: Facilitation of non-nutritive and nutritive sucking endurance and effectiveness.

Objectives and Documentation

- ♦ To increase sucking endurance. *Observe number of sucks per minute across 10-15 minute interval of PAL opportunity.*
- ♦ To increase feeding rate when nippling. *Divide number of cc of nippled nutrition by time for consumption.*
- ♦ To develop sucking bursts of 10-12 sucks before pause. *Count number of sucks between pauses.*
- ♦ To reduce pain perception through NNS release of endorphins. *Observe sucking duration and behavioral indices of pain during and following painful procedures.*

Infant Criteria

- ♦ Infant should be medically stable and have begun gavage feedings for use of PAL to affect sucking rate and sucking bursts. Infants demonstrating apnea, early fatigue, and frantic, short sucking bursts followed by fatigue would be candidates for PAL procedures to lengthen sucking pattern. Infants of 34 weeks GA or greater who are still receiving gavage feeding would be candidates for PAL procedures to increase feeding rate.
- ♦ Infants who are deemed medically able to be given a pacifier following painful procedures would be candidates for the PAL procedure to teach NNS sucking for pain relief.

Daily Nursing Approval

All PAL procedures will require daily approval of the infant's primary nursing caregiver.

Selection of Auditory Stimuli

For pacification and pain relief, selection variables are the same as for MT Intervention I. For reinforcement to increase sucking endurance across time, and for feeding benefits, music should be slightly more alerting to continue attracting the infant's attention. Again, lullabies convey important language information and are the music of choice.

Music Volume

Music volume should be set at approximately 60-65 dB (Scale C) on the PAL or 1 bar line on the machine's read out.

Music Duration

A PAL opportunity should be given 10-15 minutes once or twice/day depending on the GA of the infant. The PAL should be withdrawn when the infant ceases to suck for 1 minute with mild stimulation of pacifier movement in his/her mouth or when signs of overstimulation are observed.

Procedures

For pain relief, set pressure criteria at lowest level, set music reinforcement for 10 seconds, set suck criteria at 1, and select pacifying music. Place PAL pacifier in infant's mouth. If the infant fails to suck, stimulate sucking reflex by moving pacifier in and out of mouth gently or stroke the cheek.

For sucking endurance, set pressure criteria at lowest level initially and gradually increase, set music reinforcement for 10 seconds, and set suck criteria at 1 initially and gradually increase to desired burst level of 10-12. Gradient increments in PAL criteria for music reinforcement should only be made if infant is sucking consistently and shows progress achieving new criteria. If infant is not successful at the higher criteria, return to previous setting and allow infant a short period of success before ending the PAL opportunity for that day. Continue PAL opportunities until infant demonstrates periods of 10-15 minutes of NNS and feeding improves. This usually occurs within 1-2 days.

Infants with neurological damage or failure to demonstrate a suck reflex should be given longer periods of time at the lowest criteria for music reinforcement. Duration of reinforcement should be slightly shorter than the infant's initial rate of sucking. For instance, if the infant sucks only once/minute, then reinforcement should be set at 50 seconds.

---

[1]The PAL will be commercially available as the Sondrex P.A.L. System, from Healing HealthCare Systems, www.healinghealth.com.

Research on Music and Multimodal Stimulation

Research has shown that stimulation techniques such as skin-to-skin contact and NNS for preterm infants can offset some of the adverse neurological effects of prolonged hospitalization (Brazelton & Nugent, 1995; Britt & Myers, 1994; Gomes-Pedro et al., 1995; Harrison, 1985; Oehler, 1993; Rauh et al., 1987; Schaefer, Hatcher, & Barglow, 1980; White-Traut & Tubeszewski, 1986). Benefits from these forms of supplemental stimulation have resulted in weight gain and increased motor development (Burns, Cunningham, White-Traut, Silvestri, & Nelson, 1994). There is concern that prolonged intensive care may be detrimental to the preterm infant's intellectual development due to disruption of normal bonding and learning activities. Personnel in the NICU have become concerned that the nurturing forms of stimulation are both noncontingent and nonreciprocal. The lack of cause/effect learning may have lifelong implications for intellectual development (Burns et al., 1994).

At the intermediate stage of neonatal intensive care, there is still critical concern for the medical needs of the infant and developmental needs related to growth. Occupational Therapists facilitate feeding and neurological organization of the infant. Mothers are encouraged to bond via "kangaroo" care (holding the infant on their chest, skin-to-skin). Infants also receive "cuddling" from volunteers. Caution of overstimulation is paramount in all of these activities to avoid eliciting hypersensitive responses which disrupt neurological development (Leonard, 1993). Procedures for using music therapy techniques in infant stimulation have been previously described to promote development following hospital discharge (Standley, 1991). Research on the use of music to promote developmental gains during intermediate care in the NICU is just beginning.

One study tested a music therapy protocol for pacification, stimulation, and reinforcement of infant acquisition of developmental behaviors (Standley, 1998). Sensory, social, and motor skills were included, specifically visual and aural attending, social bonding with caregivers, differentiated vocal responses, and reaching/grasping motor behavior (Burns et al., 1994). Quiet singing served as the initial stimulus to calmly contact and pacify the infant prior to systematic addition of multiple stimuli.

Subjects for this study were 40 infants who met the following project entry criteria: (a) AGA of at least 32 weeks, (b) birth age >10 days, and (c) weight >1700 grams. Two groups, experimental and no-contact control, were matched on the basis of gender, birthweight, gestation age at birth, and severity of medical complications and each contained 10 females and 10 males.

The multimodal stimulation sequence was provided for 15-30 minutes, one to two times/week, from the time of referral by the nursing staff to discharge. Infants were cuddled, then sung to for 30 seconds without other stimulation. In the absence of distress responses, the stimulation continued with the sequential addition of cephalocaudal/proximal distal touching, rocking, and eye contact. Any physiological changes or distress responses resulted in the termination of all stimulation while disengagement cues resulted in a 15-second pause, then another trial of the stimulation. Overt pleasure responses such as snuggling, cooing, prolonged eye contact, and finger grasping were reinforced. Dependent variables were (a) days to discharge, and (b) weight gain/day.

For experimental infants, tolerance for stimulation was also assessed. These scores ranged from 1-42 computed as follows:

- 1 point for tolerated stimulation to each of 11 body sites within 15 minutes. Tolerance across two entire sequences of stimulation in 30 minutes resulted in double points.
- 1 point for intermittent infant responses of pleasure and 2 points for constant infant responses of pleasure on each of five items observed during a 15-minute stimulation sequence. These points could also be doubled if the infant demonstrated pleasure responses throughout a second sequence.

Table 9. Multimodal Stimulation Results

	Total Hospital Days		**Daily Weight Gain**	
	Male	*Female*	*Male*	*Female*
Music	55.4	32.3*	18.2 g	17.8 g
Control	56.9	44.2*	16.0 g	12.3 g

*Indicates significance ($p<.05$).

Results are shown in Table 9. Female music/multimodal stimulation subjects left the hospital significantly sooner, an average of 11.9 days earlier than the no-contact control females ($p<.05$, $df=9$, $t=2.81$). Weight gain data were not significantly different between groups.

The total length of hospitalization data are differentiated by gender. Caine (1992) found similar gender differences for discharge data in her study playing recorded music in the incubators of premature infants. Infant tolerance to stimulation across time showed that all 20 infants in the experimental group received at least three multimodal stimulation interactions and most of the females were discharged immediately thereafter. The male infants made steady, but slower, progress than females and required more intervals of stimulation prior to discharge.

A second study teaching parents the music and multimodal procedure showed that parents used the procedure, increased their visitation time in the NICU, and felt empowered to enhance their child's development (Whipple, 2000). These parents were able to use the procedure without overstimulating their child. There were also significantly fewer infant stress behaviors exhibited and significantly more appropriate parent interactions.

MT Intervention III:
Music and Multimodal Stimulation

Goals: Faciliation of neurological growth and development

Objectives and Documentation

- ♦ To increase tolerance to stimulation and homeostasis. *Record number of items in stimulation sequence completed before observance of disengagement cues. Record positive infant responses.*
- ♦ To teach parents a method of goal-oriented interaction while avoiding overstimulation of infant. *Observe parents interacting with child and appropriate use of technique. Record frequency of NICU visits and interactions.*
- ♦ To hasten readiness for discharge. *Record days to discharge.*

Program Criteria

- ♦ Infant should have achieved 30-32 weeks GA and be considered ready for minimal levels of stimulation.
- ♦ Parents who are wary of interaction with their child or those who have been observed to overstimulate their infant.

Daily Nursing Approval

♦ This procedure will require daily approval of the nurse providing care to the individual infant.

Procedures

♦ Follow procedures for the stimulation sequence below. Note that stroking should be slow, repetitious and firm since light touch is hyper-alerting to the premature infant.

AUDITORY/TACTILE/VISUAL/VESTIBULAR STIMULATION SEQUENCE (adapted with permission from Burns et al., 1994)

1. **Auditory only-30 seconds (begin with quiet humming of lullaby)**
2. **Maintain auditory and add rocking for 30 seconds**
3. **Begin tactile (stroking, then light massage) in the following order:**
   - Scalp - linear
   - Back - linear
   - Back - circular
   - Throat - linear
   - Arms - linear or circular
   - Abdomen - linear
   - Linea alba - linear
   - Legs - linear or circular
   - Cheeks - linear
   - Forehead - linear
   - Nose to ears - linear
4. **Maintain auditory and rocking and repeat tactile steps with engagement cues of eye contact and finger contact.**
5. **Note any of the following infant responses and reinforce:**
   - Head orientation
   - Smiling
   - Eye contact
   - Vocalization
   - Snuggling

ADVERSE PHYSIOLOGICAL CHANGES

1) Oxygen saturation drops below 86%
2) Heartrate <100, >200, or >20% over baseline
3) Respiratory rate >20 over baseline
4) Observed Apnea/bradycardia

Response: If any one of the above occurs, **pause 15 seconds**,
Then if HR/RR is within normal limits, **continue**. If not, **stop and consult nurse** and discontinue all stimulation for the day.

DISENGAGEMENT CUES

Subtle disengagement cues: hiccoughs, grimace, clinched eyes, eyes averted, tongue protrusion, finger splay, struggling movement

Response: Softer auditory and, if needed, pause 15 seconds.
If cue abates, continue stimulation at beginning of sequence.

Potent disengagement cues: crying, whining, fussing, cry face, spitting/vomiting, hand in halt position

Response: Offer containment and, if needed, pause 15 seconds. When cue abates, continue.

Form reprinted with permission of *Pediatric Nursing* (Standley, 1998).

In the intermediate area of the NICU in the last 2-3 weeks prior to discharge, the infant can tolerate and will benefit from greater variety and developmental challenges. Infants who remain in the intermediate NICU or in the Pediatric Intensive Care Unit beyond 40 weeks AGA are particularly in need of developmental challenges which can be effectively provided by music therapy as per established infant stimulation procedures and medical considerations.

MT Intervention IV:
Infant Stimulation

Goals: Facilitate infant alertness and response to people and the environment.

Objectives and Documentation

- To increase snuggling and cuddling responsivity. *Observe infant head orientation to holder, rooting responses, or movement of head against holder.*
- To increase eye contact with family and NICU personnel. *Observe duration of eye contact.*
- To stimulate non-crying vocalizations. *Observe vocalizations and identify content (grunts and squeaks, vs. vowels or consonants. Measure duration and frequency, attend to pitch matching of infant with auditory stimuli.*
- To increase head turn response to auditory stimuli and tracking. *Observe head orientation to site of auditory stimuli remembering in the mature infant there is a 8-11 second delay from awareness to actual head turn.*
- To increase focus and tracking of visual stimuli. *Observe as above.*

Infant Criteria

- Infant 32 weeks GA or greater and has successfully completed PAL and multimodal stimulation program, or
- Infant's status close to discharge from NICU.

Procedures

- Swaddle and hold infant in snuggle position approximately 10-12 inches from the face. Arouse infant to quiet alert state. Use infant-directed, live, slightly stimulating music to interact. Reinforce any responses included in objectives above.
- To facilitate head turn and auditory tracking, alternate input by two different people on each side of the infant or use recorded music provided via a speaker which can be moved from one side to the other of the infant's head.
- To facilitate visual focus, alternate quiet input from a variety of people in different positions about the infant (parents, siblings, medical staff, etc.).
- Discontinue any stimulation that elicits disengagement cues.

Many parents of premature infants endure anxiety, stress, and trauma related to the critical needs of their child. Parents may feel that the premature birth is somehow their fault and experience guilt. Others have hospital phobia or intimidation and do not wish to visit or interact in the NICU environment. Other parents simply have too few resources to support the extreme costs and time commitments of dealing with the needs of a premature infant. Counseling is often helpful and music therapy is a highly effective, non-threatening methodology for expression of feelings, clarification of values, identification of choices and decisions, and inspiration to act.

MT Intervention V:
Parent Counseling

Goals: Facilitate parents' comfort and relationship with their infant, his/her condition, and NICU personnel and procedures.

Objectives and Documentation

- ♦ To promote bonding and goal-oriented interactions with infant. *Record number of visits and type of interactions.*
- ♦ To assist with difficult decisions and adjustment to traumatizing issues concerning the welfare of their child. *Elicit self-report measures of emotional adjustment, stress, and comfort with decisions made.*
- ♦ To facilitate relationships with medical providers during difficult procedures. *Elicit self-report measures of perceived relationships.*
- ♦ To teach child development skills and timelines and identification of emergence of developmental delays. *Evaluate parent ability to discuss child developmental milestones and indications of infant delay.*

Referral

Referral of the interdisciplinary team caring for the infant is necessary for this procedure in order to assure adequate communication for service delivery.

Procedure

Use of standard MT counseling procedures.

Weaning From Respirator. It has also been shown that for oxygenated infants, weaning from the respirator to unaided breathing, is stressful and elicits extensive distress symptoms (Field, 1987). Music played at 60 beats/minute during weaning procedures may be indicated for respiratory regularity and increased oxygen saturation. This research is currently in progress.

Research on Music and Head Circumference Growth

Many claims have been made about the benefits of music on children's development with little research substantiation. A frequently cited proof has been the fact that school children enrolled in music education demonstrate higher scores on standardized tests and higher academic grades (Cutietta, 1996). However, researchers have long cautioned against undue attribution of these scholastic achievements to benefits of music study since a causal relationship between the two has never been established.

Recent psychological research, however, has found an intriguing increase in intellectual ability of young children following music study. Specifically, preschoolers receiving a semester of private keyboard lessons demonstrated greater long-term spatial-temporal ability on intelligence tests than did students in control conditions (Gromko & Poorman, 1998; Rauscher et al., 1997). These studies have been widely cited as emerging evidence that music may directly affect neurological development and capability, especially of young children who undergo periodic growth spurts.

Growth is critical and problematic for the premature infant and exposure to music during neonatal intensive care seems to have potential for a variety of benefits. It was recently speculated that if music promotes neurological development in infants, this might be apparent through measures of head circumference (HC), especially those taken during the infant's stay in neonatal intensive care.[2]

As a result of the rapidly growing brain, HC expands quickly in the third trimester (Guo, Roche, Chumlea, Casey, & Moore, 1997).

---

[2]This theory was first proposed by Fred J. Schwartz. M.D. during discussion at the Neonatology Research Meeting of the International MusicMedicine Conference, July 12, 1998, Royal Children's Hospital, Melbourne, Australia.

Therefore, HC of premature infants is measured regularly for determination of well being (Sutter, Engstrom, Johnson, Kavanaugh, & Ifft, 1997). Head circumference is also considered a valid indicator of brain size and intracranial volume (Buda, Reed, & Rabe, 1975). Head circumference growth during neonatal intensive care is directly correlated with long-term neurological development, especially motor skills (Forslund & Bjerre, 1990; Sommerfelt, Ellertsen, & Markestad, 1996).

Premature infants are born below the mean for HC and do not "catch up" as they mature (Sheth, Mullett, Bodensteiner, & Hobbs, 1995). The greatest deficits are apparent in the first 14 days of life. Unfortunately, the devastating deficits in HC cannot be overcome through supplemental nutrition without exceeding metabolic and renal tolerances (Berry, Conrod, & Usher, 1997). Neonatologists have cited a need for other ways of enhancing HC growth.

Research on the effects of music to benefit neurological growth during the final trimester of development is currently in progress. The possibility that a benign intervention such as music might enhance growth is exciting, though yet unsubstantiated. Since head circumference is indicative of intracranial volume and well-being, even the smallest possibility that music might enhance HC growth during neonatal intensive care and later in the child's development is particularly intriguing and merits thorough investigation.

References

American Academy of Pediatrics. Committee on Environmental Health. (1997). Noise: A hazard for the fetus and newborn. *Pediatrics*, 100(4), 724-727.

Anderson, G., & Vidyasagar, D. (1979). Development of sucking in premature infants from 1 to 7 days post birth. *Birth Defects: Original Article Series*, 15(7), 145-171.

Bernbaum, J., Pereira, G., Watkins, J., & Peckham, G. (1983). Nonnutritive sucking during gavage feeding enhances growth and maturation in premature infants. *Pediatrics*, 71(1), 41-45.

Berry, M. A., Conrod, H., & Usher, R. H. (1997). Growth of very premature infants fed intravenous hyperalimentation and calcium-supplemented formula. *Pediatrics*, 100(4), 647-653.

Brazelton, T., & Nugent, J. (1995). *Neonatal Behavioral Assessment Scale* (3rd ed.). London: Cambridge University Press.

Britt, G., & Myers, B. (1994). The effects of Brazelton Intervention: A review. *Infant Mental Health*, 15(3), 278-292.

Buda, F. B., Reed, J. C., & Rabe, E. F. (1975). Skull volume in infants: Methodology, normal values, and application. *American Journal of Diseases in Children*, 129, 1117-1174.

Burns, K., Cunningham, N., White-Traut, R., Silvestri, J., & Nelson, M. (1994). Infant stimulation: Modification of an intervention based on physiologic and behavioral cues. *Journal of Obstetric, Gynecologic, and Neonatal Nursing*, 23(7), 581-589.

Burroughs, A., Asonye, U., Anderson-Shanklin, G., & Vidyasagar, D. (1978). The effect of nonnutritive sucking on transcutaneous oxygen tension in noncrying, preterm neonates. *Research in Nursing and Health*, 1(2), 69-75.

Caine, J. (1992). The effects of music on the selected stress behaviors, weight, caloric and formula intake, and length of hospital stay of premature and low birth weight neonates in a newborn intensive care unit. *Journal of Music Therapy*, 28(4), 180-192.

Cassidy, J. W., & Ditty, K. M. (1998). Presentation of aural stimuli to newborns and premature infants: An audiological perspective. *Journal of Music Therapy*, 35(2), 70-87.

Cassidy, J. W., & Standley, J. M. (1995). The effect of music listening on physiological responses of premature infants in the NICU. *Journal of Music Therapy*, 32(4), 208-227.

Chapman, J. S. (1979). Influence of varied stimuli on development of motor patterns in the premature infant. In G. Anderson & B. Raff (Eds.), *Newborn behavioral organization: Nursing research and implications* (pp. 61-80). New York: Alan Liss.

Coleman, J. M., Pratt, R. R., Stoddard, R. A., Gerstmann, D. R., & Abel, H. (1997). The effects of the male and female singing and speaking voices on selected physiological and behavioral measures of premature infants in the intensive care unit. *International Journal of Arts Medicine*, 5(2), 4-11.

Collins, S. K., & Kuck, K. (1991). Music therapy in the Neonatal Intensive Care Unit. *Neonatal Network*, 9(6), 23-26.

Cutietta, R. A. (1996). Language and music programs. *General Music Today*, 9(2), 26-31.

DeCasper, A. J., & Carstens, A. A. (1981). Contingencies of stimulation: Effects on learning and emotion in neonates. *Infant Behavior and Development*, 4, 19-35.

DeCasper, A. J., & Fifer, W. P. (1980). Of human bonding: Newborns prefer their mothers' voices. *Science*, 208, 1174-1176.

Detterman, D. (1978). The effect of heartbeat sound on neonatal crying. *Infant Behavior and Development*, 1, 36-48.

DiPietro, J., Cusson, R., Caughy, M., & Fox, N. (1994). Behavioral and physiologic effects of nonnutritive sucking during gavage feeding in preterm infants. *Pediatric Research*, 36(2), 207-214.

Field, T. (1987). Alleviating stress in intensive-care unit neonates. *Journal of American Obstetrical Association*, 9, 129-135.

Field, T., Ignatoff, E., Stringer, S., Brennan, J., Greenberg, R., Widmayer, S., & Anderson, G. (1982). Nonnutritive sucking during tube feedings: Effects on preterm neonates in an intensive care unit. *Pediatrics*, 70(3), 381-384.

Flowers, A., McCain, A., & Hilker, K. (1999). *The effects of music listening on premature infants.* Paper presented at the Biennial Meeting, Society for Research in Child Development, Albuquerque, NM.

Forslund, M., & Bjerre, I. (1990). Follow-up of preterm children: II. Growth and development at four years of age. *Early Human Development*, 24(2), 107-118.

Gardner, S. L., Garland, K. R., Merenstein, S. L., & Lubchenco, L. O. (1997). The neonate and the environment: Impact on development. In G. B. Merenstein & S. L. Gardner (Eds.), *Handbook of neonatal intensive care* (pp. 564-608, 4th ed.). St. Louis: Mosby.

Gill, N., Behnke, M., Conlon, M., McNeely, J., & Anderson, G. (1988). Effect of nonnutritive sucking on behavioral state in preterm infants before feeding. *Nursing Research*, 37(6), 347-350.

Goff, D. M. (1985). The effects of nonnutritive sucking on state regulation in preterm infants. *Dissertation Abstracts International*, 46(8-B), 2835.

Gomes-Pedro, J., Patricio, M., Carvalho, A., Goldschmidt, T., Torgal-Garcia, F., & Monteiro, M. (1995). Early intervention with Portuguese mothers: A 2-year follow-up. *Journal of Developmental and Behavioral Pediatrics*, 16(1), 21-28.

Gordin, P. C. (1990). Assessing and managing agitation in a critically ill infant. *MCN*, 15, 26-32.

Gorski, P., Davison, M., & Brazelton, T. (1979). Stages of behavioral organization in the high-risk neonate theoretical and clinical considerations. *Seminars in Perinatology*, 3(1), 61-72.

Gromko, J. E., & Poorman, A. S. (1998, July). *The effect of music training on preschoolers' spatial-temporal task performance.* Paper presented at International Society for Music Education, Johannesburg, South Africa.

Guo, S. S., Roche, A. F., Chumlea, W. C., Casey, P. H., & Moore, W. M. (1997). Growth in weight, recumbent length, and head circumference for preterm low-birthweight infants during the first three years of life using gestation-adjusted ages. *Early Human Development*, 47, 305-325.

Harrison, L. (1987). Effects of early supplemental stimulation programs for premature infants: Review of the literature. *Maternal-Child Nursing Journal*, 14, 69-90.

Hill, A. (1992). Preliminary findings: A maximum oral feeding time for premature infants, the relationship to physiological indicators. *Maternal-Child Nursing Journal*, 20(2), 81-92.

Kanarek, K., & Shulman, D. (1992). Non-nutritive sucking does not increase blood levels of gastrin, motilin, insulin and insulin-like growth factor 1 in premature infants receiving enteral feedings. *Acta Paediatrica Scandinavica*, 81(12), 974-977.

Leonard, J. E. (1983). Music therapy: Fertile ground for application of research in practice. *Neonatal Network*, 12(2), 47-48.

McCain, G. (1992). Facilitating inactive awake states in preterm infants: A study of three interventions. *Nursing Research*, 41(3), 157-160.

McCain, G. (1995). Promotion of preterm infant nipple feeding with nonnutritive sucking. *Journal of Pediatric Nursing*, 10(1), 3-8.

Medoff-Cooper, B., & Gennaro, S. (1996). The correlation of sucking behaviors and Bayley Scales of Infant Development at six months of age in VLBW infants. *Nursing Research*, 45(5), 291-296.

Moore, R., Gladstone, I., & Standley, J. (1994, November). *Effects of music, maternal voice, intrauterine sounds and white noise on the oxygen saturation levels of premature infants.* Paper presented at the National Association for Music Therapy, Inc., National Conference, Orlando, FL.

Oehler, J. (1993). Developmental care of low birth weight infants. *Advances in Clinical Nursing Research*, 28(2), 289-301.

Palmer, M. M. (1993). Identification and management of the transitional suck pattern in premature infants. *Journal of Perinatal and Neonatal Nursing*, 7(1), 66-75.

Rauh, V., Nurcombe, B., Achenbach, T., & Howell, C. (1987). The mother-infant transaction program: An intervention for the mothers of low-birthweight infants. In N. Gunzenhauser

(Ed.), *Infant stimulation: For whom, what kind, when, and how much?* (Pediatric Round Table Series: 13). Skillman, NJ: Johnson & Johnson Baby Products.

Rauscher, F., Shaw, G., Levine, L., Wright, E., Dennis, W., & Newcomb, R. (1997). Music training causes long-term enhancement of preschool children's spatial-temporal reasoning. *Neurological Research*, 19(1), 2-8.

Rybski, D., Almli, C., Gisel, E., Powers, J., & Maurer, M. (1984). Sucking behaviors of normal 3-day-old female neonates during a 24-hr period. *Developmental Psychobiology*, 17(1), 79-86.

Schaefer, M., Hatcher, P. & Barglow, P. (1980). Prematurity and infant stimulation: Review of research. *Child Psychiatry and Human Development*, 10(4), 199-212.

Schunk, H. A. (1993, November). *The relationship between background music during feeding time and weight gain of low-birthweight infants: A pilot study.* Unpublished study presented at National Association for Music Therapy, Inc., National Conference, Toronto, Canada.

Schwartz, R., Moody, L., Yarndi, H. & Anderson, G. (1987). A meta-analysis of critical outcome variables in nonnutritive sucking in preterm infants. *Nursing Research*, 36(5), 292-295.

Sheth, R. D., Mullett, M. D., Bodensteiner, J. B., & Hobbs, G. R. (1995). Longitudinal head growth in developmentally normal preterm infants. *Archives of Pediatric and Adolescent Medicine*, 149(12), 1358-1361.

Sommerfelt, K., Ellertsen, B. & Markestad, T. (1996). Low birthweight and neuromotor development: A population based, controlled study. *Acta Paediatrica*, 85(5), 604-610.

Standley, J. (1991). The role of music in pacification/stimulation of premature infants with low birthweights. *Music Therapy Perspectives*, 9, 19-25.

Standley, J. (1998). The effect of music and multimodal stimulation on physiologic and developmental responses of premature infants in neonatal intensive care. *Pediatric Nursing*, 24(6), 532-538.

Standley, J. (2003). The effect of music-reinforced non-nutritive sucking on feeding rate of premature infants. *Journal of Pediatric Nursing*, 18(3), 169-173.

Standley, J., & Moore, R. (1995). Therapeutic effects of music and mother's voice on premature infants. *Pediatric Nursing*, 21(6), 509-512, 574.

Standley, J. M. (1996). A meta-analysis on the effects of music as reinforcement for education/therapy objectives. *Journal of Research in Music Education*, 44(2), 105-133.

Standley, J. M. (2000). The effect of contingent music to increase non-nutritive sucking of premature infants. *Pediatric Nursing*, 26(5), 493-495, 498-499.

Stelmachowicz, P. G. (2000). Amplification for infants. *Seminars in Hearing*, 12(4), 409-422.

Sutter, K., Engstrom, J. L., Johnson, T. S., Kavanaugh, K., & Ifft, D. L. (1997). Reliability of head circumference measurements in preterm infants. *Pediatric Nursing*, 23(5), 485-490.

Whipple, J. (2000). The effect of parent training in music and multimodal stimulation on parent-neonate interactions in the Neonatal Intensive Care Unit. *Journal of Music Therapy*, 37(4), 250-268.

White-Traut, R., & Tubeszewski, K. (1986). Multimodal stimulation of the premature infant. *Journal of Pediatric Nursing*, 1(2), 90-95.

Woodson, R., & Hamilton, C. (1988). The effect of nonnutritive sucking on heart rate in preterm infants. *Developmental Psychobiology*, 21(3), 207-213.

Yeh, T. F., Voora, S., & Lilien, D. (1980). Oxygen consumption and insensible water loss in premature infants in single- versus double-walled incubators. *Journal of Pediatrics*, 97, 967-971.

Zahr, L. K., & Balian, S. (1995). Responses of premature infants to routine nursing interventions and noise in the NICU. *Nursing Research*, 44, 179-185.

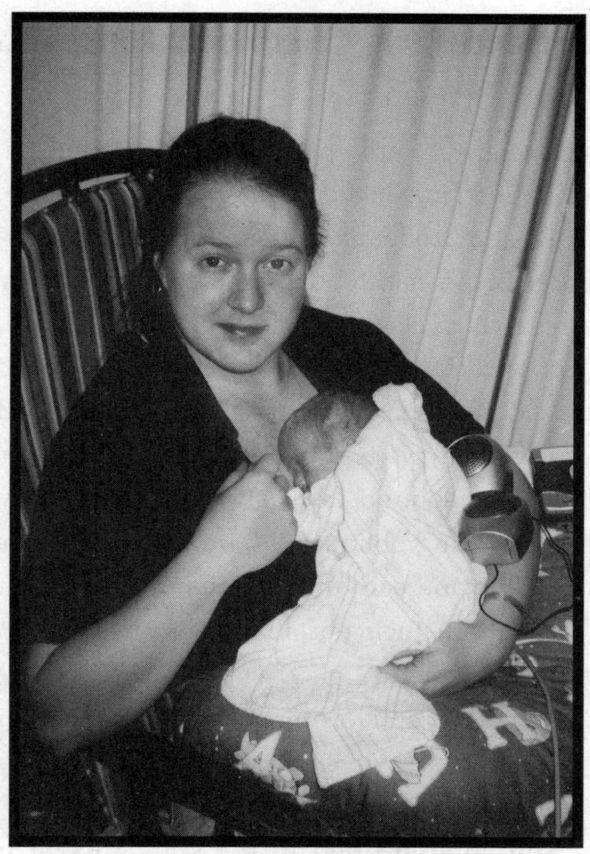

After almost three months in the NICU, Libby and Nikki enjoy quiet music together at home at last.

4 | Infant and Early Childhood Music Therapy

Music Therapy in early childhood is the specialized use of music by qualified music therapists to teach developmental, social, pre-academic, and academic skills to infants, toddlers, and at-risk pre-K children and to teach bonding, training, and parenting skills to their parents. A qualified Music Therapist is an individual with national certification from the Certification Board for Music Therapists, as designated by the initials MT-BC. Music therapy early childhood services may be provided in hospital neonatal intensive care units, as homebound instruction, in community daycare or service settings, or in public school programs. Children are eligible for music therapy and early intervention from birth through age 5 years or throughout their enrollment in pre-K school programs, including those who are:

1. Premature and low birth weight infants beginning life in neonatal intensive care.
2. Students with a developmental disability.
3. Students enrolled in the state's Early Intervention Preschool Program.
4. Infants at-risk of developmental delay or disability due to medical reasons, exposure to abuse or toxic substances, residence in foster care, migrant or homeless status, assessment as marginal for exceptional child education or being economically disadvantaged.

Increased survivability of lower birth weight infants contributes to the incidence of disabilities in the population of children who will require special educational and medical services. Long-term studies have shown that as low birth weight children mature, they continue to require medical care. They are twice as likely to be hospitalized during the ages of 3-5 years and will spend longer in the hospital than will normal birth weight children. The most common medical problems encountered are asthma, upper and lower respiratory infections, and ear infections. Additionally, growth attainment is decreased (Hack, Klein, & Taylor, 1995).

During the school years, children born prematurely are 50% more likely to be enrolled in special education programs and are more likely to repeat a grade during school. A small percentage will be diagnosed with mental retardation and/or cerebral palsy while most will evidence milder cognitive, focus of attention, and neuromotor functioning deficits (Hack et al., 1995).

The most common neurological problem of children born prematurely is cerebral palsy with incidence increasing as birth weight decreases: normal birth weight = <5% incidence; between 2500 and 1500 grams = 6-8% incidence; between 1500 and 1000 grams = 14-17% incidence; under 1000 grams = 20% incidence (Hack et al., 1995). There is also a higher incidence of behavior problems that increases as birth weight decreases. This is especially true for males.

Long-term follow-up of premature children attaining adulthood shows that their quality of life and self-image is equivalent to that of persons born as term infants (Tideman, Ley, Bjerre, & Forslund, 2001). In only one area is there a discernible difference. A greater proportion of those born prematurely have lifelong physical health complications than do those born at term.

Identifying Long-term Developmental Disabilities

Long-term developmental disabilities are often not evident until months after discharge and are difficult to distinguish from immature, but typical, infant behavior. Therefore, constant monitoring and referral for detection of developing problems are essential. Parents, medical professionals and early intervention specialists all contribute to this monitoring/referral process so that specific early intervention services can be provided as soon as the need becomes apparent. It has been clearly established that early intervention improves long-term outcomes in learning, education, and overall development and is most effective when started as early as possible. It should be noted that early intervention programs are less effective in ameliorating neuro-developmental outcomes than educational or health issues. Because of the high risks, some parents do not wait for a developmental delay to be diagnosed but immediately enroll their premature infants in special infant stimulation prevention programs.

In Figure 7, developmental problems are listed by typical post-birth age at which delays are usually noticeable. It should be noted that each infant develops according to his/her individual genetic and environmental factors. Therefore, timelines are approximate and screening for developmental delays should consider all factors in a child's life, including home or daycare environment, family history of child development, gestational age at birth, life experiences and opportunities.

Developmental Timeline for the First Two Years

Assuming no acquired sensory deficits, at the time of discharge from the NICU, the premature infant's sensory abilities approximate those of a term infant. The infant's vision is the least sophisticated sense with visual acuity at 20 feet being equivalent to that of an adult at 400-600 feet. Objects 10 inches away are clearest to the

Emergence of Developmental Delays*

At 6 months:
- attachment disorder, failure to bond
- eye-hand coordination problems in handling objects or self-feeding
- failure to develop basic language interactions such as cooing or babbling
- hearing loss identified by failure to startle or attend to sound, diminished cooing, lack of response to parent's voice.

Between 6-12 months:
- visual impairments; retinopathy of prematurity (ROP)
- cerebral palsy
- moderate to severe mental handicap
- hearing loss evidence by failure to respond to waving hello or good-bye, failure to track sound, failutre to listen to music/TV, failure to babble or use consonant sounds

At 12 months:
- minor neurological dysfunction evident in coordination or memory
- hearing loss (5% of premature infants born <32 weeks gestational age)

At 18 months:
- slight cerebral dysfunction and learning problems
- attention deficits
- language problems

At 3 years:
- mild mental handicap
- behavioral problems, hyperactivity

Between 3-6 years:
- learning difficulties

Between 6-9 years:
- specific learning disabilities

*Adapted from *What to Do When Your Baby Is Premature* by Joseph A. Garcia-Prats, M.D. and Sharon G. Hornfischer, RN, BSN, copyright©2000 by Joseph Garcia-Prats, M.D. and Sharon G. Hornfischer, RN, BSN. Used by permission of Three Rivers Press, a division of Random House, Inc.

Figure 7. Emergence of Developmental Delays

newborn. The sense of touch is advanced, with the infant using body movement to convey acceptance or discomfort due to changes on the skin such as a puff of cool air versus the warm breath of a parent when cuddled under the chin. The sense of smell is sophisticated enough for the infant to recognize his/her mother. Taste preferences for sweets are already apparent. The infant will use all of the senses

Table 10. Developmental Timeline for the First 2 Years

Age	Motor and Perceptual Development	Language Development	Social and Personal Development
Term birth - 40 gestational weeks	• *Startles, cries, or awakens to loud sounds • Responds to auditory stimuli • *Responds to visual stimuli with high contrast colors held 9-12" from face • Responds to tactile stimuli • Flexes and extends arms and legs	• Demonstrates differentiated crying, fussing	• Self-regulates behavioral states
1 month	• Attends to auditory, visual, and tactile stimuli • Lifts head momentarily • Demonstrates hand to mouth coordination • Move arms to midline	• *Alerts to name	• Crying ceases when held and soothed • Smiles • Recognizes caregiver • Interacts in quiet, alert state
2 months	• *Tracks auditory and visual stimuli with focused attention • *Turns head to parent's voice • *Recognizes familiar stimuli • Moves arms past midline • Lifts head when held on shoulder	• Makes cooing, vowel sounds	
3-4 months	• Lifts head when on stomach • Grasps and moves object • Reaches toward object • Balances head in supported, sitting position • Bears some weight on legs	• *Signals needs such as "pick me up" • Laughs	• Vocalizes with interactions. • Matches sung pitches • Reacts to peek-a-boo
5-6 months	• Rolls over-stomach to back • Sits up momentarily • Crosses midline with grasp and release of object • Rolls over-back to stomach • Holds own bottle • Finger feeds self a cracker	• Makes babbling sounds, imitates speech sounds • Looks for source of novel sound, notices toys that make sounds • Responds to "no" or change in parent's voice • Vocalizes with inflection	• Soothes self with thumb or pacifier • Mimics • Reciprocates passing objects to others • Opens mouth for spoon

Table 10 continued. Developmental Timeline for the First 2 Years

Age	Motor and Perceptual Development	Language Development	Social and Personal Development
7-8 months	• Pulls up to stand • Stands alone • Finger feeds with pincer grasp • Scoots/crawls • Sits in high chair	• Looks at labeled objects • Shows awareness of changing stimuli • Attends to TV • Shows preference for and interest in words with 1st syllable accent • Matches pitches of simple melody with step-wise, descending intervals *(Three Blind Mice)*	• Plays peek-a-boo • Laughs and squeals with delight
9-10 months	• Sits alone • Creeps well • Walks holding on with reciprocal leg motion	• Listens when spoken to • Says "MaMa, DaDa, Bye-Bye"	• Plays pat-a-cake
11-12 months	• Walks • Drinks from a cup • Uses finger to point to an object	• Responds to simple requests like, "Come here" • Recognizes words for common objects • Moves objects in beat to music	• Amuses self for short periods • Plays independently • Indicates wants with point or vocalization • Attends to read or sung information
12-18 months	• Climbs stairs • Feeds self with spoon	• Demonstrates 20-40 word vocabulary • Sings songs without words	• Uses 2-word phrase • Follows simple directions
18 months - 2 years	• Imitates gross motor skills such as hopping, jumping, marching, etc.	• Learns to label 2-5 new objects/day • Combines 2 words into a phrase	• Toilets when a scheduled opportunity is given • Shares • Participates in simple conversation • Holds hand of adult to walk to aspecific destination, through parking lots, etc. • Scribbles on paper

*Denotes key behaviors indicating ability to see and hear.

to learn from the environment and develop. Major developmental milestones are indicators of progress and their attainment carefully evaluated through the first 3-5 years of life.

Screening for major problems is accompanied by detailed, ongoing assessment of the child according to developmental accomplishments in the first two years of life. Table 10 is a compilation of milestones taken from the research literature in child development, linguistics, and music education. Asterisks on the chart denote key behaviors indicating ability to see and hear and allow for constant screening of the child's progress in developing these key abilities for learning. Again, actual timelines are normative approximations and can vary widely among children. A substantial deviation from the norm is necessary for an actual diagnosis of a specific developmental delay.

Children born prematurely are assessed for developmental delay according to corrected age, not chronological age. Corrected age is their gestational age at birth plus months of life, not their chronological birthday forward. For instance, an infant born at 32 gestational weeks by Dubowitz evaluation who is now 2 months old chronologically would be evaluated for functioning at a newborn level since 32 weeks plus 8 weeks equates to 40 weeks or term birth for a newborn. At 6 months of age, this child would be evaluated according to developmental milestones for a 4 month old infant.

Stimulating Language Development

Language is the most critical developmental skill for facilitating all learning activities. It is imperative to promote and reinforce it from birth. All individuals interacting with the infant should learn to identify and respond in a timely fashion to the infant's developing awareness and use of speech and language concepts. Following are general guidelines for promoting language development:

- Girls are usually 1-2 months ahead of boys on language development milestones. Child development charts provide a basic guideline for when skills are usually developed but are not exact for any particular child. Remember that steady progress through the items is more critical than trying to force a child to have a skill by a particular date.
- Follow the infant's lead. Mimic and enthusiastically respond to the infant's vocalizations and interactions. Shape or model the sound to the closest word approximation. Do not pressure the child to produce a sound or word.
- Talk in running commentary about your activities. It is important to talk to the child in live interactions frequently and control the amount of time spent in non-live listening such as listening to television and recorded media. Around 4 months of age, the infant is ready for "conversations" without the use of actual words. At this age the infant will make eye contact and reciprocate vocalizations demonstrating the ability to take turns in conversing by pausing for the other person to speak. This is a good time to mimic and shape the infant's vocalizations.
- Speak in correct language, not baby talk. Use the pronoun I instead of referring to yourself in the third person.
- Speak slowly and distinctly to the child. Use a lot of face-to-face contact.
- Play interactive games such as Peek-a-Boo and Pat-a-Cake.

- When the child begins to talk, do not correct his/her language; rephrase it. If the child says "ba" and points to a cookie, respond with "Oh, you want a cookie."
- Touch or point to what you talk about. Also guide the child in touching and pointing to what you are talking about. Reinforce eye contact with the object. When the infant looks at something, say, "Oh, you are looking at the ________."
- Encourage taking turns during talking to teach conversational concepts.
- Sing often to the child. Babies are fascinated by music from birth. Changes in tempo, pitch and volume are alerting. Monotony in pitch, tempo and volume are soothing. Parents can compose their own music for singing about everyday activities.
- Use rhymes. Children are fascinated by rhyming sounds.
- Use surprise. Children are very alert to novel sounds.
- Use language in context with the environment or interaction and focus on the positive. For instance, say hello to greet a child awakening from sleep instead of making a complaining comment about the child's crying upon awakening.
- Expand the child's utterances. If the child says, "dog," then say, "You see a dog." Link concepts together by adding additional sentences, such as, "The dog wants to come inside."
- Place an emphasis on language in the context of daily routine. Read the infant a book every night before bed to promote literacy and to link language with literacy.

Early Intervention Resources

Enrichment, early intervention, and special education programs were funded in 1975 with Public Law (P.L.) 94-142 and again in 1986 when P.L. 99-457 extended special education programs to qualified children ages 3 to 5 years. Section H of this law provided early intervention for disabled infants birth to 2 years. These programs have been available now for 10 years and demonstrate excellent success. Low birth weight infants receive special services after discharge from the hospital and many will have disabilities requiring such services through adolescence. Still, the medical costs far outweigh the educational costs related to this problem with the cost of initial hospitalization being the greatest expenditure (Lewit et al., 1995). Programs such as music therapy which shorten hospitalization and increase developmental skills in the hospital are a desirable developmental training intervention. Continued early intervention following discharge is essential in enrichment and prevention of developmental delay.

Music therapy procedures have proven effective with premature, developmentally disabled, and at-risk infants, toddlers and preschool children. It enhances early intervention to maximize individual potential and prevent further developmental delays. In fact, research has demonstrated that music therapy procedures utilized by qualified music therapists have resulted in:

- Shortened hospital stays and developmental gains for premature infants in neonatal intensive care.
- Increased developmental gains in children in Early Intervention programs.
- Increased pre-reading and pre-writing skills in children in Early Intervention programs.
- Increased developmental, social, and academic gains in children in Exceptional Student Education programs.

Music Therapy and Infant Stimulation

Music Therapists are adept at infant stimulation. Music can be combined with other sensory input to foster developmental gains in sensory, social, and motor skills. Following are examples of music activities to teach a specific developmental skill for the ages birth through 2 years. Active engagement in all activities is more effective for learning than is passive listening. Infants attend to music more fixedly than to other stimuli. These music activities are developmentally appropriate and provide opportunities for active engagement, sensory integration, and the initiation of social encounters.

Developmental Music Activities

Birth

Music for Sleeping

- Select a specific piece of music to accompany sleeping and play/sing it with soft vocalizations every time child is put down to sleep. Combine it with other soothing stimuli such as swaddling, dim lighting, non-nutritive sucking, or gentle rocking. A lullaby is designed to soothe and is an excellent selection. You might consider *Hush Little Baby, Brahms' Lullaby, All the Pretty Little Horses, Rock-a-Bye Baby, When You Wish Upon A Star.*

Music for Alerting

- Select a specific music for alerting the infant to your approach and play/sing it each time infant awakens and you wish to start an interaction. A hello song for this purpose also incorporates the language concept of greeting. Consider *Hello, Hello, How Do You Do? Hello, Everybody.*

Music for Tactile Awareness and Habituation

- Cuddle infant and sing a quiet lullaby while firmly, but gently, massaging down the body from the head to the back, then the chest to the legs. If infant startles to any part of his/her body being touched, stop the massage in that area and return to an area higher up the body. Avoid a light touch which is discomforting to the infant's immature neurological system. The child's neurological system develops from the top down and massage will enhance tolerance to touch. Give guided assistance to enable the infant to place his/her hands in the mouth for exploration.

Music for Vestibular Stimulation

- Select quiet music with very stable rhythm. Gently and slowly rock the infant in various planes and positions: to and fro, up and down, side to side. Do not invert the infant during this movement. Observe the infant for indications of overstimulation such as grimacing, nystagmus, crying, arms and legs widely extended and, if observed, stop immediately. Continue to rock quietly to soothe the infant. This activity may be done while the child is lying down with the child rocked from prone to sidelying. As the child progresses, swings, rocking chairs, waterbeds, and gently moving gymnastic balls may be added.

1 month

Music for Auditory/Visual Tracking

- Assure that the infant is in a quiet, alert state. The Music Therapist and partner should sit on each side of the baby lying supine on floor. One sings, waits for infant to turn head, then enthusiastically interacts with infant. Then, the partner sings, waits for infant to turn head to the other side, and enthusiastically interacts. Remember to give the infant plenty of time to respond since the neurological system is still immature. For some infants, this may require up to 5 seconds. The infant hears higher pitches best, so sing in higher keys. Consider the songs, *What is Your Name?, This Is What I Can Do.*

- With child and therapists in the same position as above, center an object approximately 12" above the child's face. Wait for the child's eyes to fixate on it, then slowly move it to one side then the other in time to slow, calm background music. The object must be red or black-white contrast (such as a bull's eye) for the child to see it clearly.

Music to Stimulate Hand to Hand Exploration

- Select and play background music. Hold the infant's arms so that the hands are together. Move them slowly in time to music so that the infant can explore the hands palm to palm, moving around each other, or tapping together.

2 months

Music to Stimulate Vowel Sounds

- Assure that infant is a quiet, alert state. Face infant about 10 inches away and say, "oohhh." Use facial affect to reinforce attention to your face, approximations of mouth to circular shape, and any vocalizations.
- Assure that infant is in a quiet, alert state. Face infant and slowly chant vowel sounds in singsong style with accentuated mouth movements, as in chorus of *Old McDonald* (*ee, i, ee, i, o*) or sounds like "ooo-ee-ooo-ee-ohh." Respond enthusiastically to any vocal sounds and mimicry of mouth shapes. Mimic the baby's responses.

Music for Interaction

- Sing *If You're Happy and You Know It, SMILE* and accompany with exaggerated facial affect. Change smile to hug and accompany with physical affection such as hugging. Use similar procedure for kissing. Music and approach to infant should be quiet and gentle so that the infant will not be startled. Respond enthusiastically if infant smiles or vocalizes.

2-3 months

Music for Movement

- Place infant supine on cookie tray. Slide the tray gently on the carpet to recorded music, such as a waltz. Use back and forth and side to side motions.
- Hold the infant with his/her back to your chest then dance to recorded music. Turn, sway, and dip to music.
- Place infant prone on floor and sit in front of him/her. When the child lifts his/her head, make eye contact and start singing. When the head drops, cease the music immediately. Continue using music to reinforce head control. As the infant gains head control, music can be used similarly to reinforce turning the head to the side.
- Give the infant a rattle that is easily grasped. Sing in time with infant's shaking of the rattle. Cease singing when the infant drops the rattle or stops shaking it. Music will reinforce grasp and rhythmic movement of the rattle.

Music for Mother-Infant Attachment

- Hold and cuddle the infant when in a quiet alert state. Look in his/her eyes. Stroke the face or hair gently. Sing a lullaby with the word *Mother* used repeatedly. This can be an original composition as a gift for your baby. If you do not feel that you can make up a song, simply put new words to a simple melody like *Three Blind Mice* or *Twinkle, Twinkle Little Star*. Just be sure that the word *Mother* is repeatedly used.

Singing to Stimulate Pitch Matching in Vocalizations

- Sing children's songs to infant and notice any pitch matching when infant vocalizes. Mimic the infant's vocal responses. Consider *ABC Song; Hot Cross Buns; It's Raining, It's Pouring.*

4 months

Music to Stimulate Babbling

- Compose a MaMa song, a repetitive melody that uses the word *MaMa* and an interaction in each line and accompany the singing with the action, i.e.,

  MaMa loves _____*(baby's name)* while hugging infant
  MaMa touches ______ while stroking infant's face
  MaMa tickles _______ while gently tickling stomach.
  Respond to the infant's vocalizations and mouth movements approximating the "mmmm" sound.

- Compose a similar, but different song for every member of the infant's family, i.e., *Here Comes Joey* for a big brother.

Music for Social Interaction

- Two adults sit on the floor across from each other with the baby between legs of one, back to adult chest. Roll a ball back and forth to music. Several infants or small children can participate if each is assisted by an adult. Simply enlarge the circle.
- Form an infant music group with adults standing in circle each holding an infant with back to the adult's chest. Dance to recorded music with approach to center of circle, then backing up. Turn around to music. Weave in and out of the circle. When the approach toward center is

made, let babies touch each other briefly. Move smoothly and slowly so that infants will not startle. For each movement, allow several beats before movement changes.

Music to Stimulate Hand to Knee Behavior

- Place infant in supine position. Bend the knees with the feet flat on the floor. Give guided assistance with the arms so that the hands reach the knees. Tap the knees to music. For variety, stop tapping and stretch arms and legs out with massage, then go back to knee tapping with flexed knees.

Music to Stimulate Pointing

- Hold the child with his/her back to your chest. Give guided assistance with one hand with the finger free "to point." Use a singsong, rhythmic chant with animated inflections while walking around the room pointing to all the objects: "This is a chair. A what? A chair! ... This is a door. A what? A door! ... This is a window. A what? A window! ... etc.

5 months

Music to Stimulate Listening

- Sing songs with surprise sounds such as *Pop Goes the Weasel* and use a vocal surprise "POP" by placing finger in mouth. Sing a song about a train such as *Little Red Caboose* and make chugging sounds or simulate a train whistle. Sing a song about birds such as *Blue Bird* and simulate a bird call. Sing a song about a cat or dog and simulate a meow or barking sound. Objects that whistle, click, pop, clack, flutter, etc. are perfect for this activity. Assure that the sung material provides a context for the sound such as singing about a train and then hearing its sound. Respond to infant's response to surprise sound.

Music to Stimulate Hand to Foot Behavior

- Place infant in supine position. Flex the pelvis. Give guided assistance with the arms so that the hands reach the feet. Tap the feet to music and help the infant explore his/her toes. For variety, stop tapping and stretch arms and legs out with massage, then go back to foot exploration.

6 months

Music for Moving in Rhythm

- Prop or hold the infant sitting up. Play recorded music with strong beat (march, dance). Give infant an object that is small enough to be grasped and makes a sound when shaken... bells, egg shaker, infant rattle.
- Play recorded music and allow child to bang unbreakable pots and pans with wooden spoons.

Music to Reinforce Reading Concepts

- Obtain books that are also songs, such as *Eensy, Weensy Spider* or *Twinkle, Twinkle, Little Star.* Read the book and point to the pictures. Sing the words and point to the pictures.

Music for Rhyming

- Sing chants that rhyme such as:

  ________*(name) or MaMa points to the door*
  ________*(name of the infant) looks at the door*
  ________*(name) or MaMa points to the floor*
  ________*(name of the infant) looks at the floor.*

  Accompany singing with the activity.

- Sing songs such as *Hickory, Dickory Dock; A Tisket, A Tasket; Eensy, Weensy Spider; One, Two, Buckle My Shoe.*

7-8 months

Musical Hide and Seek

- Use a variety of objects and a scarf. Sing

  I see the _______ (point to the object)

  Where did it go? (Cover the object with the scarf)

  Peek-a-boo!! (Whip the scarf off).

Music to Stimulate Singing

- Face the child and hold his/her hands. Sing and clap well known children's songs such as *Baa, Baa, Black Sheep; Old King Cole; London Bridge; Clap, Clap, Clap Your Hands; Head, Shoulders, Knees and Toes; She'll Be Coming 'Round the Mountain; Are You Sleeping?; Bingo; This Old Man; The Wheels on the Bus; Put Your Finger on Your Nose; Hokey-Pokey; Paw-Paw Patch; Skip to My Lou.* Respond enthusiastically to all "singing" vocalizations.

Music for Independent Play

- Play a recorded, extended length album. Give child several objects that make noise. Let the child entertain him/herself.

1 year

Music to Label Objects

- Use a simple, repetitive melody which can be a well-known one, borrowed for this purpose. Sing:

  I see a _______ (object)

  I see a ________ (different object).

- Hold the child and dance around, touching each object named. Let the child touch the object when it is approached.

Music for Following Directions

- Sing songs with directions, such as

  Clap your hands, stomp your feet

  Turn around, take your seat.

- Sing, *Put your hands on your head, on your head* naming various body parts or *Get your toy and come here, come here, come here to me.*

Music for Blowing

- Give child a safe toy that makes music when blown. (A kazoo, plastic recorder, or large whistle are too large to be swallowed and have no removable parts that can pull off and be inhaled.) Model blowing the object to produce noise. When the child imitates, reinforce this newfound ability. Model rhythmic sounds or humming sounds to accompany a song.

Music for Scribbling

- Give toddler large crayon and paper. Sing a scribble song:

  Scribble up and down and all around

  Write a message to Mother

  Send the scribble home with the child and suggest that the family place it on refrigerator, referring to it often and telling the infant, "You wrote a message to Mother." Teach infant to scribble only on the paper. Put the crayon away when unsupervised.

References

Garcia-Prats, J., & Hornfischer, S. (2000). *What to do when your baby is premature.* New York: Three Rivers Press.

Hack, M., Klein, N., & Taylor, H. (1995). Long-term developmental outcomes of low birth weight infants. *The Future of Children* [On-line serial], 5(1). Available: http://www.futureofchildren.org/LBW/12LBWHAC.htm.

Lewit, E., Baker, L., Corman, H., & Shiono, P. (1995). The direct cost of low birth weight. *The Future of Children* [On-line serial], 5(1). Available: http://www.futureofchildren.org/LBW/12LBWHAC.htm.

Tideman, E., Ley, D., Bjerre, I., & Forslund, M. (2001). Longitudinal follow-up of children born preterm: Somatic and mental health, self-esteem and quality of life at age 19. *Early Human Development*, 61, 97-110.

Glossary of Medical and Developmental Terms

ABR—abbreviation for auditory brainstem response test. See brain stem auditory evoked response.

Adjusted gestational age (AGA)—the estimated age in weeks of a fetus or newborn from conception to current date. It is based on the infant's due date, calculated as 40 weeks from the onset of the mother's last menstrual period or on a Dubowitz assessment completed at birth.

AGA—see adjusted gestational age and appropriate for gestational age.

Anencephaly—a genetic anomaly that can be detected early in the pregnancy by amniocentesis or ultrasonography and is incompatible with survival, in which large portions of the brain are missing and the brainstem is malformed.

Anomaly—an abnormality.

Anoxia—lack of oxygen resulting from deficient oxygen supply to the respiratory system, failure of the blood to carry oxygen to the tissues, or failure of the tissues to absorb oxygen. Cerebral anoxia refers to lack of oxygen in the brain.

APGAR evaluation—a score of 0 to 10 given at birth and again 5 minutes after birth to assess the infant's physical well-being and immediate need for resuscitation. With repeated low scores, the assessment may continue to be repeated every 5 minutes, as deemed appropriate. The score is based on heart rate, respiratory effort, muscle tone, reflex irritability, and color. Infants with 5 minute scores of 7 and higher have much better neurologic outcomes than infants with lower scores. Scores of 8 and higher require no support, scores of 4-7 usually result in resuscitation, and scores lower than 4 require intubation for the infant's survival.

Apnea—the absence of spontaneous respiration, lasting at least 15-20 seconds.

Appropriate for gestational age (AGA)—neonate of typical size and maturation based on length of gestation, regardless of pre-, full-, or post-term delivery.

Arterial blood gas—a blood sample taken from an artery, usually through an umbilical line, to measure acid-base balance, ventilation related to carbon dioxide, and oxygenation.

Arterial catheter—a thin plastic tube inserted in an artery to draw blood or measure blood pressure.

Asphyxia—the absence of blood flow and oxygen resulting in loss of consciousness and potential death, requiring immediate provision of oxygen and artificial ventilation in order to prevent brain damage.

Aspiration—can refer to either suctioning material from the body or inhaling a substance, such as meconium, formula, or stomach contents into the lungs, which can lead to aspiration pneumonia.

At-risk infant—child with developmental condition or problem that may have significant impact on future functioning. This designation qualifies the child for early intervention services.

Audiometric testing—a comprehensive hearing evaluation consisting of air and bone conduction testing and speech testing. Used to determine hearing thresholds, sound discrimination, and word recognition abilities.

Auditory brainstem response (ABR)—a test of an infant's hearing acuity in which brain waves are measured in response to various auditory stimuli in order to determine the existence and type of hearing loss.

Auditory threshold—the lowest level of intensity at which a sound is perceived.

Awareness—voluntary or involuntary response to sensory stimulation.

BAER—see brain stem auditory evoked response. Test performed to diagnose nervous system abnormalities and hearing losses by focusing on changes in brain waves stimulated by a clicking sound.

Bagging—a procedure used to temporarily assist an infant's respiration; oxygen is provided via compression of an air bag attached to a small mask placed on the infant's face.

BID (also bid, BD, bd)—an abbreviation meaning twice daily.

Bilirubin—a bile substance that is orange-yellow in color, is produced by the breakdown of red blood cells, and normally travels through the bloodstream to the liver where it is excreted into bile.

Blood urea nitrogen (BUN)—blood test that measures kidney and liver function based on blood urea and nitrogen.

Bonding—the reciprocal attachment process between the infant and parents, also referred to as maternal-child attachment, which affects psychological and physical development of the infant. In normal infants, bonding begins immediately after birth when the infant is placed on the mother's abdomen. Eye contact and embrace of the infant close to the parent's body are important factors in establishing positive attachment.

BPD—see bronchopulmonary dysplasia.

Bradycardia—a heart rate below 100 beats per minute (for infants).

Brain bleed—see intraventricular hemorrhage and intracranial hemorrhage.

Brain stem auditory evoked response (BAER)—the first 10 milliseconds of electric brainstem activity following the introduction of an auditory stimulus, for which 7 peaks would indicate normal hearing, a delayed response could indicate middle or inner ear disorder hearing loss, and fewer than 7 peaks could indicate a neural disorder.

Breastfeeding—the act of feeding the infant milk directly from the mother's breast, facilitated by the infant sucking the breast, also referred to as nursing.

Bronchopulmonary dysplasia (BPD)—the condition, also called chronic lung disease, that may develop following long-term artificial or assisted pulmonary ventilation, in which the lungs and bronchioles lose elasticity, lung tissue is scarred, and pulmonary arterial walls thicken

BUN—see blood urea nitrogen.

Burping—the releasing of gas from the stomach through the mouth, facilitated in the infant by stroking and tapping the infant's back periodically during and following feeding.

Cardiopulmonary resuscitation (CPR)—for infants, an emergency life support procedure consisting of artificial respiration and manual external cardiac massage in which the infant's mouth and nose are covered by a mask or by the caregiver's mouth for introduction of small breaths of air. The tips of 2 or 3 fingers placed on the infant's midsternum and lined up with the nipples are used to provide compressions of ½ to 1 inch, resulting in 5 compressions alternated with one ventilation at a rate of 100 compressions and 20 ventilations per minute.

Cause/effect relationship—the relationship between observed behavior or response of an infant (effect) and the immediately preceding event (cause) in the environment which stimulated it.

Central line—an intravenous line threaded through a vein until it nears the heart, providing continuous access for introduction of fluids and medications and gathering of diagnostic data. Establishment of a central line ensures accessibility in the event of peripheral vein collapse.

Central nervous system (CNS)—the brain and spinal cord, responsible for processing information to and from the nerves of the body and regulating and coordinating the body's functions, including sleep, muscle movement, hunger and thirst.

Central venous catheter—flexible catheter inserted into the tip of the superior vena cava. Used to obtain blood samples.

Cephalocaudal development—the head to toe progression of infant neurological maturation.

Cerebral palsy (CP)—see developmental disabilities associated with prematurity.

Cerebrospinal fluid (CSF)—fluid flowing through the brain and spinal column, protecting four ventricles, subarachnoid spaces, and spinal canal and assisting in controlling breathing based on changes in carbon dioxide levels.

Cesarean section—the surgical delivery of an infant through an incision through the mother's abdomen and uterus when abnormal fetal or maternal conditions exist that indicate potential danger for a vaginal delivery.

Chest physiotherapy (CPT)—the use of cupping or manual percussion and vibration to loosen and move mucus and fluids from the lungs so that expectoration by coughing and suctioning can occur. Cupping entails tapping the patient's affected lung and bronchial areas with a cupped hand. Vibration is created by tension and contraction of the caregiver's hand, arm, and shoulder while the same hand is placed on the patient's affected lung or bronchial area as the patient exhales, increasing the movement of exhaled air within the small bronchi.

Chest tube—a catheter inserted through an incision into the chest cavity to release air, allowing a collapsed lung to re-expand.

Chronic lung disease (CLD)—see bronchopulmonary dysplasia.

Circumcision—a commonly performed surgical procedure under local anesthesia, in which the foreskin of the newborn male's penis is removed to prevent potential infection. Some religious beliefs support ritual circumcision.

CLD—see chronic lung disease.

Corticosteroid—a steroid produced by the adrenal cortex.

CNS—see central nervous system.

Co-bedding—the practice of placing multiple birth infants (e.g., twins, triplets, etc.) together in one radiant warmer, incubator, or open crib to approximate familiar intrauterine conditions, providing the infants require the same type of bedding based on clinical stability and ability to control body temperature and that one infant does not have an infection that could be transmitted to another.

Cognition—the mental process associated with perception, thought, reason, and memory.

Colic—intestinal discomfort without specific determined cause, often marked by crying.

Colostomy—a surgical opening allowing the colon to empty its contents into a bag through the abdominal wall.

Colostrum—yellow fluid consisting of maternal antibodies, white blood cells, water, protein, fat, minerals, vitamins, and carbohydrate secreted by the breast during the first few days following delivery prior to the beginning of lactation.

Continuous positive airway pressure (CPAP)—pressurized air, which can be accompanied by additional oxygen, delivered to the infant with the purpose of keeping the lungs expanded while the infant inhales and exhales.

Corrected gestational age (CGA)—see adjusted gestational age.

Cortisol—a steroid hormone produced naturally in the body. Its release is indicative of stress.

CP—see cerebral palsy.

CPAP—see continuous positive airway pressure.

CPR—see cardiopulmonary resuscitation.

CPT—see chest physiotherapy.

Crying—a sudden, loud, voluntary or automatic vocalization that is part of a fear, pain, or startle response. Can also indicate hunger or desire for attention.

CSF—see cerebrospinal fluid.

CVC—see central venous catheter.

dB—see decibel.

D/C—an abbreviation either meaning discontinue, such as to D/C a particular medication or feedings, also abbreviated as d/c, DC, dc, and disc; or meaning discharge, such as to D/C from the hospital, also abbreviated d/c, DC, and disch.

Decibel (dB)—unit of measure of intensity (loudness) of a sound stimulus.

Desaturation—occurrence of a decreasing degree to which oxygen is bound to hemoglobin, expressed as a percentage of the total possible saturation limit.

Developmental tests of infant ability

Alberta Infant Motor Scales—measures infant motor development and maturation from birth to 18 months of age.

Bayley Scales of Infant Development—psychomotor assessment for infants aged 1-42 months.

Neonatal Behavioral Assessment Scale (NBAS)—developed by Brazelton to assess infant ability to respond to the environment and provide recommendations for caregiving, especially for disorganized infants unable to respond to or hypersensitive to stimuli. The 28 observable behaviors include habituation to light, rattle, bell, and tactile stimulation of the foot; orientation to auditory and visual stimuli; level of alertness, irritability, and activity; frequency of smiles and startles; skin color; general muscle tone; and reflexes of rooting and sucking.

Peabody Developmental Motor Skills—Assesses infants from birth-5 years of age on gross and fine motor skills to determine need for special education. The testing kit has remediation suggestions for problems identified.

Developmental disabilities associated with prematurity

Attention deficit disorder (ADD)—a condition related to central nervous system functional deficits without detectable anomalies, characterized by short attention span, limited concentration, and often hyperactivity.

Cerebral palsy (CP)—a disorder in motor functioning appearing before the age of 3 years caused by permanent, nonprogressive brain damage present from birth or soon after. Usually associated with premature or abnormal birth and intrapartum asphyxia resulting in damage to the central nervous system, CP abnormalities and delays may be evident in breathing, sucking, swallowing, speech, responsiveness, and limb movement, including walking.

Epilepsy—a group of neurologic disorders characterized by one or more of the following: convulsive seizures, sensory disturbances, and loss of consciousness.

Hearing impairment—limitation in a person's hearing ability that challenges his/her ability to communicate.

Hyperactivity—a condition characteristic of inattention, distractibility, difficulty organizing tasks and sequencing activities, and excessive movement, for which there is an increased incidence among premature infants due to neurologic immaturity at birth.

Mental retardation (MR)—disorder in which both intelligence and environmental functioning and adaptation abilities are below average.

Minimal brain dysfunction (MBD)—see attention deficit disorder above.

Specific learning disability (SLD)—one of many disorders of basic psychological processes in understanding or using language, e.g., inability to read, write, spell, or do mathematics. Does not include learning problems due to specific visual, motor, or hearing handicaps or other identifiable developmental disabilities.

Visual impairment—limitation in a person's hearing ability that challenges his/her ability to function.

Discrimination—a learned difference in responding to the presence of two stimuli, one of which is reinforcing and therefore emits a response, the other of which is not reinforcing and therefore is ignored.

Disengagement cues—signs displayed by the infant that indicate overstimulation, including yawning, hiccoughing, sneezing, tongue protrusion, finger splay or outstretched arm, struggling movements, clinched or averted eyes, change in skin color, grimacing, moro reflex, wide-eyed fixed stare, crying or cry face, spitting or vomiting, irregular heart rate or respiration rate, oxygen desaturation, or limp body and lack of responsiveness. Overstimulation interrupts neurological maturation. Therefore, when the infant emits these signs, he/she should be placed in a crib in a quiet, dim room and left alone to rest.

Diptheria and tetanus toxoids and pertussis vaccine (DTP or DPT)—an active immunization routinely administered to children under 6 years to protect against diptheria, tetanus, and pertussis (whooping cough).

DPT (also DTP)—see diptheria and tetanus toxoids and pertussis vaccine.

Dubowitz—assessment of the infant's physical development, completed at birth in order to estimate gestational age, which closely resembles progress toward the due date, but can suggest accelerated or retarded intrauterine development.

Ductus arteriosis—a blood vessel in the fetus joining the descending aorta and the pulmonary artery, which normally closes after birth, but may not be closed in premature infants. It often requires medical treatment or surgery in order to facilitate necessary flow of blood and oxygen to the lungs.

Due date—projected date of birth for a pregnant woman, also referred to as estimated date of confinement (EDC), calculated as 40 weeks from the onset of the mother's last menstrual period.

Dyslexia—a language processing impairment affecting the ability to read due to difficulty discriminating left from right and letter and word sequences.

Early intervention—the identification and delivery of comprehensive services to children with special needs from birth and includes those with disabilities and those at-risk.

Echocardiogram—a graph of heart activity created from ultrasound.

EDC—abbreviation for estimated date of confinement. See due date.

Edema—swelling due to accumulation of fluid in body tissue.

EEG—see electroencephalogram.

EKG (also ECG)—see electrocardiogram.

Electrocardiogram (ECG or EKG)—a graph of electrical heart activity detected through leads attached to the patient's chest, used to diagnose cardiac abnormalities.

Electroencephalogram (EEG)—a graph of brain waves, labeled alpha, beta, delta, and theta rhythms based on the frequencies they produce, detected by electrodes placed on the scalp.

Electrolytes—elements that dissociate into ions when dissolved in another solvent, such as water, and are able to conduct electric current. Balance is necessary for proper metabolism and physical functioning.

Electronic fetal monitor (EFM)—a device for the electronic evaluation of fetal heart rate response to movement, external stimuli, and uterine contractions. Measurement may occur externally or internally.

Endotracheal tube—a large-bore airway catheter inserted through the nose or mouth, through the larynx, and into the trachea to deliver oxygen under pressure in cases of general anesthesia and when total control of ventilation is required.

Epilepsy—see developmental disabilities associated with prematurity.

Episiotomy—an incision is made into the perineum and then sutured following delivery to facilitate delivery and prevent tearing of the perineum.

Estimated date of confinement (EDC)—see due date.

Exchange transfusion—exchange of 75 to 85% of the infant's blood with whole blood to treat hemolytic anemia or hyperbilirubinemia.

Extubation—removal of the endotracheal tube.

Fetal alcohol syndrome (FAS)—set of physical, behavioral, and psychological characteristics that often appear in infants of mothers who consumed alcohol during pregnancy, including low birth weight and intrauterine growth retardation, central nervous system and cardiovascular abnormalities, cognitive deficits, and craniofacial abnormalities, such as small head, low set ears, folds and cracks around small eyes, crossed eyes, short nose, large forehead, and small chin.

Fine motor skills—abilities involving the coordination of small muscles (e.g., muscles of the hand).

Flaccid tonus—weak, soft muscle tone.

Flexion—generally, a movement of the human skeleton that decreases the angle between two adjoining bones. In birth, the bending of the neck of the fetus so that the chin nears the chest, which occurs as a result of resistance as the fetus travels through the birth canal.

Fontanel—the space between the unconnected sections of the baby's skull, also referred to as the soft spot.

Full term (FT)—gestation between 37 and 42 weeks at birth.

FT—see full term.

G tube—see gastrostomy device.

GA—see gestational age.

Gastroesophageal reflux (GER)—the backflow of acidic stomach contents into the esophagus, producing burning sensation in the esophagus.

Gastrointestinal tract (GI)—the muscular tube, also referred to as digestive tract, extending from the mouth to the anus, including the pharynx, esophagus, stomach, and small and large intestines.

Gastrostomy device (G tube)—a catheter inserted directly into the stomach following gastrotomy with the purpose of providing nutrition and administering medication.

Gastrostomy—a surgically created opening to the stomach on the external abdominal wall, the procedure for which is called gastrotomy.

Gavage feedings—the provision of nutrition through a nasogastric or orogastric tube used when the infant has a weak or uncoordinated sucking response or frequent apneic episodes.

Genetics—the study of heredity based primarily on the chromosomal makeup of the human body.

GER—see gastroesophageal reflux.

Gestational age—the age of the fetus measured in weeks from the onset of the mother's last menstrual period prior to conception.

GI—see gastrointestinal tract.

Germinal matrix hemorrhage (GMH)—most common type of brain bleed that occurs in the mass of embryonic cells over the caudate nucleus that is present only in the fetus.

GMH—see germinal matrix hemorrhage.

Grasp reflex—the inward flexing of fingers or toes in response to stroking of the palm of the hand (palmar grasp reflex) or sole of the foot (plantar grasp reflex).

Gravida—referent for a pregnant woman, for which the first pregnancy is delineated by gravida 1 or primagravida, the second is notated as gravida 2 or secundigravida, etc.

Gross motor skills—abilities involving the coordination of large muscles to accomplish generalized tasks (e.g., walking).

Habituation—sensory or physiologic acclimation to a stimulus.

Healthy Start—a screening and referral service provided by Florida law since 1991 to improve birth outcomes through improved prenatal and perinatal care.

Heart rate monitor—see monitors.

Heel stick-procedure—also referred to as heel puncture, in which a sample of blood is obtained from the infant's heel for testing.

Hematocrit—the percentage of red blood cells in the blood.

Hernia—an intestinal protrusion through the muscular tissue of the abdominal wall, potentially leading to tissue death; umbilical and inguinal hernias, appearing at the naval and groin, respectively, are most common in neonates.

High-risk—referent either for a patient, especially an infant within the first 28 days of life, who has an elevated chance of poor outcome or for status of the patient in a Level III neonatal or newborn intensive care unit.

HMD—see hyaline membrane disease.

Homeostasis—internal balance of the physiologic systems, including heart beat, respiration, blood pressure, and body temperature, that operate together to maintain proper body function.

Hyaline membrane disease (HMD)—respiratory distress caused by a lack of surfactant in the lungs, also referred to as respiratory distress syndrome.

Hydrocephalus—an abnormally large accumulation of cerebrospinal fluid in the ventricles of the brain, resulting from improper drainage of the ventricles, leading to increased intracranial pressure.

Hyperactivity—see developmental disabilities associated with prematurity.

Hyperaldosteronism—a disease caused by excess production of the normal adrenal hormone, aldosterone. It causes high blood pressure and low serum potassium.

Hyper-alert—excessive awareness of sensory stimuli, physically manifested in muscle tension, wide-eyed stare, and physiologic and visceral responses.

Hyperbilirubinemia—abnormally high level of bilirubin in the blood, also referred to as jaundice, that may result in lethargy, yellowing of the skin and eyes, and changes in visceral responses, as well as dangerously high levels that can result in kernicterus. Treatment entails phototherapy, increased hydration, and, if necessary, umbilical blood transfusion.

Hypoxia—state of decreased oxygen.

Ileostomy—surgical creation of an opening through the external abdomen to the small bowel to allow the passage of stool when the lower bowel functions inadequately.

ICH—see intracranial hemorrhage.

Incubator—environmentally controlled enclosed infant bed for protection and temperature maintenance.

Infant states or levels of awareness:

Crying—awake state with fussing, wailing, or yelling by infant to communicate needs such as hunger, discomfort, or desire for attention.

Active alert—awake state in which infant makes frequent rhythmic movements of the arms and legs and is usually seeking attention.

Quiet alert—awake state when infant is lying quietly, eyes open, making eye contact and exhibiting regular breathing and steady heart rate. This is the best time for interacting, teaching, or bonding with the infant.

Drowsy—an intermediate state between waking up or falling asleep.

Active sleep or light sleep—Infant is asleep with frequent moving of arms and legs, changing facial expressions, and rapid eye movement (REM). Alternates about every 30 minutes with quiet sleep state.

Quiet sleep or deep sleep—Infant is asleep and unmoving with steady heart and respiration rates. Face is relaxed. No REM.

Infusion pump—electronic apparatus that monitors and dispenses intravenous fluids and medications.

Intermediate care—special care nursery that is a step down from the intensive care or high-risk environment; the majority of the care is focused on nutritional development and growth of the infant.

Intracranial hemorrhage (ICH)—spontaneous rupture of blood vessels of the brain.

Intravenous (IV)—term for administration of fluids or medications by injection into a vein.

Intubation—insertion of the endotracheal tube.

Intraventricular hemorrhage (IVH)—spontaneous rupture of blood vessels within the brain's ventricles that occurs in 40% of premature infants, usually within the first 3 days of life. It is frequently bilateral.

Intrauterine growth retardation (IUGR)—delayed or inadequate development of the fetus in the womb.

Isolette—brand name for incubator.

IUGR—see intrauterine growth retardation.

IV—see intravenous.

IVH—see intraventricular hemorrhage.

Jaundice—see hyperbilirubinemia.

Kernicterus—neurological damage caused by a toxic level of bilirubin in the blood.

Kangaroo care—skin-to-skin contact in which the infant is placed directly on the parent's chest to promote breathing and facilitate homeostasis, growth, and parent-infant bonding.

Lactose—milk enzyme that is a component of manufactured infant formulas and is a potential allergen in infants, which would require an alternative soy-based formula.

Lanugo—soft, white, downy hair covering the entire body of the fetus from the 5th through the 9th months of gestation, and consequently present on some premature infants.

Large for gestational age (LGA)—neonate with length and weight greater than 90% of infants appropriate for gestational age, regardless of pre-, full-, or post-term delivery.

Laryngomalacia—abnormally narrow larynx resulting in restriction of respiratory function.

LBW—see low birth weight.

Level I hospital—the primary care aspects of a health care facility, including outpatient departments and well-baby care, in which early detection and prevention as well as health maintenance are the focus of care.

Level II hospital—secondary or acute care facility or hospital unit into which patients are either admitted directly or by referral, focusing on emergency and critical care, providing comprehensive diagnosis and treatment of a wide range of medical problems.

Level III hospital—tertiary care, such as the highly sophisticated and specialized units of a hospital, to which patients are referred from the primary and secondary care levels in order to receive advanced treatment for complex pathologies.

Lipids—nutritional fat provided intravenously when oral intake is contraindicated.

Low birth weight (LBW)—birth weight below 2500 grams or 5½ pounds. The infant is categorized as very low birth weight if below 1500 grams.

Lower respiratory infection (LRI)—inflammation of the larynx, trachea, lungs, bronchi, or bronchioles caused by virus or bacteria.

LP—see lumbar puncture.

LRI—see lower respiratory infection.

Lumbar puncture (LP)—the insertion of a needle and stylet between the third and fourth lumbar vertebrae, also referred to as a spinal tap, to obtain a sample of cerbrospinal fluid for the purpose of diagnosis or therapeutic drainage.

Magnetic resonance imaging (MRI)—creation of a comprehensive picture by radiofrequency radiation that provides soft tissue contrast and view of multiple plains without the radiation hazards of other types of imaging; it is used to detect any internal soft tissue abnormalities, including those of the central nervous system.

Meconium—thick, sticky, green-black substance that collects in the intestines of the fetus and forms the first newborn stools; the presence of meconium in the amniotic fluid during labor may indicate fetal distress and pose danger of infant aspiration.

Medications common in the NICU

Acyclovir—prescribed to treat herpes virus infections, including chicken pox and shingles, as well as AIDS.

Aldactone—a diuretic, for which the generic is spironolactone, that is used to treat high blood pressure, to eliminate excess body fluid, and in the diagnosis and treatment of hyperaldosteronism.

Amoxicillin—antibiotic within the penicillin family used to treat a variety of infections including gonorrhea, otitis media, skin, respiratory, urinary, and genital infections.

Ampicillin—penicillin-like antibiotic used to treat respiratory, urinary, genital, and gastrointestinal infections, gonorrhea, and meningitis, that is routinely prescribed with gentamicin for high-risk neonates.

Ampicin—see ampicillin.

Aminiphylline—see theophylline.

Amphotericin—antifungal drug for systemic infections.

Aquaphor—healing salve for skin.

Cisapride—medication used for gastroesophageal reflux or bowel preparation for colonoscopy.

Claforon—an antibiotic.

Decadron—see dexamethasone.

Demerol—an analgesic.

Dexamethasone—corticosteroid used to reduce inflammation existent with severe allergic reactions, anemias, skin and eye infections, digestive tract and lung diseases, and fluid retention related to kidney damage. It is give for cerebral edema, sepsis, and extubation.

Digoxin—a digitalis glycoside prescribed to treat cardiac problems including congestive heart failure and irregular heartbeat by improving cardiac strength leading to improved circulation and reduction of edema.

Dilantin—antiepileptic, generically called phenytoin sodium, prescribed to prevent seizures either related to a seizure disorder or following neurosurgery.

Diuril—a diuretic, known generically as chlorothiazide, used to treat high blood pressure and other conditions requiring the elimination of excess body fluid.

Dobutamine—medication used in the treatment of cardiac problems.

Dopamine—cardiotropic given for hypotension.

Drisdol—Vitamin D supplement given for jaundice.

Endecin—diuretic.

Epinephrine—drug used for resuscitation.

Erythromycin—antibiotic effective in the treatment of numerous infections, including those of the skin, eyes, and genital, urinary, gastrointestinal, and respiratory tracts.

Fentanyl—narcotic analgesic used to sedate the agitated, ventilated neonate.

Fortaz—an antibiotic.

Gentamicin—antibiotic, routinely prescribed with ampicillin for high-risk neonates, used to treat many gram-negative bacteria, such as Pseudomonas, and some gram-positive bacteria, including Staphylococcus aureus.

Indocin—see indomethiacin.

Indomethiacin—nonsteroidal anti-inflammatory prescribed to reduce inflammation, swelling, stiffness, and pain. Given for closure of patent ductus arteriosus and prevention of intraventricular hemorrhage. Also known as indomethacin.

Insulin—hormone used by the body to effectively process food, especially sugar.

Kanamycin—broad-spectrum antibiotic effective in treating specific gram-negative, gram-positive, and acid-fast bacteria.

Lasix—diuretic, generically called furosemide, used to eliminate excess fluid from the body, effective in the treatment of hypertension, congestive heart failure, liver and kidney disease, and fluid accumulation in the lungs.

Morphine—narcotic analgesic used in the management of moderate to severe pain.

Mycostatin—used for oral thrush or candida diaper rash.

Narcan—drug used for resuscitation.

Nystatin—antifungal medication used to treat skin infections.

Oxacillin—given for staphylococcal disease.

Pavulon—skeletal muscle relaxant, generically referred to as pancuronium bromide, administered to ventilated patients.

Phenobarbital—barbiturate used to aid sleep and to treat seizure disorders.

Poly-Vi-Sol—multivitamin supplement containing at least 9 vitamins.

Reglan—used to treat symptoms of gastroesophageal reflux by expediting emptying of stomach contents.

Survanta—chemical sprayed in infant's respiratory tract to prevent respiratory distress syndrome.

Tagament—given for hyperacidity or GI hemorrhage.

Theophylline—bronchial dilator used to treat symptoms of asthma, bronchitis, and hyaline membrane disease by relaxing the airway smooth muscle.

Tylenol—acetaminophen for fever, mild pain.

Vancomycin—antibiotic used to treat intestinal infections.

Vitamin D—vitamin supplement that assists in bone structure development due to its role in calcium absorption and is provided to prevent the development of rickets.

Zantac—given for hyperacidity and GI hemorrhage.

Meningitis—inflammation of the membranes surrounding the spinal cord and brain due to bacteria or virus, diagnosed using lumbar puncture. Symptoms include headache, neck stiffness, fever, irritability, and fatigue. Lasting damage can include deafness, blindness, paralysis, and mental retardation.

Meningocele—an anomaly present at birth in which the membranes surrounding the spinal cord and brain protrude through an opening in the spinal cord or skull that contains cerebrospinal fluid and can be surgically repaired.

Microcephaly—a congenital anomaly in which the head is small in relation to the rest of the body, meeting the criterion of head size more than two standard deviations below the average circumference based on length of gestation, age, gender, and ethnicity. Mental retardation results from pressure of the developing brain against the abnormally small skull, preventing complete development and causing brain damage.

Monitors

Apnea—detects changes in thoracic or abdominal movement and heart rate and sounds an alarm if breathing stops.

Blood pressure—either continuously or on a periodic basis measures and records diastolic and systolic blood pressure.

Cardiac—used for continuous observation of heart functions and may include electrocardiograph and oscilloscope readings, recording devices, and visual record of heart function and rhythm, as well as an alarm system to alert to abnormal rhythms and rates.

Cardiorespiratory—used to facilitate continuous observation of heart and respiratory rates and rhythms, to alert to any abnormalities, and also referred to as cardiac apnea monitor (CAM).

Heart rate—a device that monitors heart rhythms both audibly and by electrical wave formation and alerts to deviation from normal cardiac function.

Pulse oximeter—a clip, containing heating coils which raise skin temperature and increase blood flow at the surface, that is placed on tip of finger or band wrapped around another pulse point, such as the ankle, to measure oxyhemoglobin in the blood to evaluate oxygen saturation level.

Temperature probe—the sensor attached to the infant's skin from the incubator in order to monitor body temperature.

Transcutaneous oxygen/carbon dioxide sensor—measures the oxygen or carbon dioxide content in the blood through electrodes attached to the skin.

Moro reflex—the normal response in infants through 4 months of age, also called a startle reflex, in which a sudden loud noise or slight raising and then dropping of the infant's head results in flexion of the legs, abduction of arms, and often brief crying. Neurologically immature infants may have an exaggerated reflex and may lack the ability to reorganize themselves following the startle response, remaining in the moro reflex position.

Motor ability—skill of motion regulation, governed by muscle, nerve, or brain center in order to complete purposeful activities.

MRI—see magnetic resonance imaging.

Multisensory stimulation—stimulation of the infant, also referred to as multimodal stimulation, that occurs in a simultaneous or cumulative mode, usually consisting of auditory, tactile, visual, and vestibular stimuli.

Multiple birth—more than one infant delivered from an individual mother, as a result of one pregnancy, e.g., twins, triplets, etc.

Myelinating—development of coating of nerve fibers throughout the body.

Myopia—nearsightedness.

Nasal canula—pronged tube inserted in the nostrils for the purpose of delivering oxygen.

Naso-gastric tube (NG tube)—flexible tube inserted in one nostril and passed through the esophagus into the stomach for the purpose of gavage feeding, administration of oral medication, and release of stomach gas.

NBICU—abbreviation for newborn intensive care unit. See neonatal intensive care unit.

NBIMCU—abbreviation for newborn intermediate care unit. See intermediate care.

Nebulizer—a device that humidifies and delivers air and oxygen as well as respiratory medications.

NEC—abbreviation for necrotizing entercolitis.

Necrotizing enterocolitis (NEC)—an inflammatory disorder of the bowel in which intestinal tissue death occurs due to the attack of naturally existing bacteria on the inflamed tissue.

Neonatal intensive care unit (NICU)—special care hospital nursery unit for the care of high-risk newborns, labeled newborn intensive care unit in some hospitals (NBICU).

Neonate—description of an infant during the first 30 days of life.

Nesting—opportunity provided prior to hospital discharge for parents to further bond with their infant overnight while managing their infant's care with hospital staff supervision and support as needed. This usually occurs in a room designed as a family bedroom adjacent to the NICU.

Neurological development—progression of cephalocaudal and proximodistal central and peripheral nervous system formation and maturation.

Neurological dysfunction—anomalous development of central and peripheral nervous systems.

Neurons—the basic nerve cells of the nervous system with the purpose of impulse conduction.

Newborn intensive care unit (NBICU)—see neonatal intensive care unit.

NG tube—see nasogastric tube.

NICU—see neonatal intensive care unit.

NIMCU—abbreviation for neonatal intermediate care unit. See intermediate care.

Nippling—term used to describe bottle feeding.

NNS—see non-nutritive sucking.

Noncontingent stimuli—Environmental stimuli which occur, but are not due to, the observed behavior of the infant.

Non-nutritive sucking (NNS)—natural reflex of the infant to suck on an object not providing nourishment (e.g., thumb or pacifier) for the purpose of comfort.

Nonreciprocal stimuli—an event or stimulus in the environment that is not interactive with infant. It does not lead toward maturation. For instance, by necessity infant crying has no discernible effect on the application of a painful medical procedure.

Nothing by mouth (NBM or NPO)—term meaning that the patient is to receive no nutrition or medication orally.

NPO—abbreviation from the Latin nulla per os, meaning nothing by mouth.

Nystagmus—involuntary, rapid, rhythmic movement of the eye.

OAE—see otoacoustic emissions test.

OG tube—see orogastric tube.

Omphalocele—an anomaly allowing the intestines to protrude through an opening in the abdominal wall.

Orogastric tube (OG tube)—flexible tube inserted through the mouth and passed through the esophagus into the stomach for the purpose of gavage feeding, administration of oral medication, and release of stomach gas.

Oral—motor development-the coordination of finger to mouth exploration, as an infant first explores all objects with his/her mouth.

Orient—to attend to a stimulus by immediate focused response, e.g., turning head toward sound.

Osteopenia—condition of weak and fragile bones caused by mineral loss.

Otitis media—an inflammation of infection of the middle ear that is common in early childhood, usually following upper respiratory infection, and is treated with antibiotics, analgesics, and decongestants.

Otoacoustic emissions test—a screening test to ascertain whether newborns' inner ears are functioning. It measures the presence of vibrations produced by healthy ears.

Ototoxic—descriptor for something damaging to hearing that can refer to specific medications necessary to high-risk infant survival.

Oxygen saturation (SaO2)—the percentage of oxygen saturation in the blood, based on the binding of oxygen to hemoglobin.

Oxygen hood—a tent-like apparatus that may be placed over the head of a hospitalized neonate to deliver highly-concentrated oxygen. Sometimes referred to as an oxy-hood.

Oxytocin—a hormone that causes uterine contraction and is administered to induce or expedite labor and to control postpartum bleeding; its use can result in uterine rupture, fetal hypoxia, and jaundice.

Pacification—the process of calming and regaining homeostasis.

Palmar grasp reflex—see grasp reflex.

Para—a combining form to designate the number of viable children a woman has produced. Usually stated as para 1, para 2, etc.

Parentese—a natural way of speaking to infants, also referred to as motherese and baby talk, that typically includes decreased volume and higher pitch than normal speech, concentration on vowels, melodically fluctuating cadences, repetition, clear enunciation, and pauses between words and phrases.

Patent ductus arteriosus (PDA)—a common occurrence in premature infants in which the ductus arteriosus remains open following birth; it is repaired surgically if closure does not occur spontaneously.

PDA—see patent ductus arteriosus.

PEEP—see positive end-expiratory pressure.

Percussion and postural drainage (PPD or P & PD)—see chest physiotherapy.

Perineum—the tissue between the vagina and anus that is often torn during childbirth. Episiotomy, in which an incision is made into the perineum and then sutured following delivery, may be elected to facilitate delivery and prevent tearing.

Peripheral intravenous line—IV inserted into arm or leg which can remain for 2-4 days. It is used for short-term infusion therapy. It is also sometimes referred to as a peripheral intravenous catheter (PIC).

Periventricular leukomalacia (PVL)—morbid softening of the tissue around the ventricles of the brain that indicates poor neurological outcome.

Phototherapy—treatment for hyperbilirubinemia in which the neonate is placed under a florescent blue light with eyes and genitalia covered for protection; exposure of the neonate's bare skin to ultraviolet light accelerates the excretion of bilirubin in the skin, decomposing it by photooxidation. The infant may receive continuous treatment for several hours to several days, during which time parents and caregivers are limited in the amount of time they may remove the infant from underneath the light to facilitate bonding through holding.

Physician specialists

Anesthesiologist—a physician specializing in the administration of anesthesia for medical and surgical procedures; after completing a 4-year residency in anesthesiology, an anesthesiologist may administer anesthesia directly, supervise its delivery by a nurse anesthetist, or serve as a consultant.

Cardiologist—a specialist in diagnosing and treating heart disorders.

Endocrinologist—a physician who has completed training in the sub-specialty of internal medicine that focuses on the diagnosis and treatment of disorders of the endocrine system, including the pancreas, gonads, and the thyroid, suprarenal, adrenal, and pituitary glands.

Gastroenterologist—a physician who specializes in the diagnosis and treatment of gastrointestinal tract disorders and diseases.

Hematologist—a physician specializing in blood and blood-forming tissues.

Neonatologist—a physician who has completed training in the sub-specialty of pediatrics that focuses on the comprehensive medical treatment of newborns.

Nephrologist—a medical specialist in diagnosing and treating diseases, disorders, and dysfunctions of the kidneys.

Neurologist—a physician specializing in the diagnosis and treatment of disorders of the nervous system.

Ophthalmologist—a physician specializing in the diagnosis and treatment of eye injury, disorder, and disease.

Orthopedist—a specialist in the diagnosis and treatment of disorders of body movement, including the skeletal and muscular systems and related joints and tissues.

Pediatrician—a physician who has completed training in the development and medical treatment of children from birth through age 21.

Perinatologist—a physician specializing in the care of the mother, fetus, and neonate regarding the diagnosis and treatment of disorders developing during gestation, childbirth, and time period immediately following birth.

Pulmonologist—a medical specialist who focuses on the diagnosis and treatment of diseases and disorders of the respiratory system, specifically the lung.

PIC—abbreviation for peripheral intravenous catheter. See peripheral intravenous line.

PIE—see pulmonary interstitial emphysema.

Pinna—the external ear that assists in localization of auditory stimuli.

PIP—see pulmonary insufficiency of the premature.

Pitch—the frequency of vibrations of an auditory stimulus. Infants begin to match vocal pitches by the age of 3 months.

Plantar grasp reflex—see grasp reflex.

Pneumothorax—the collection of air in the pleural space between the lungs and ribs that causes lung collapse, treated by insertion of a chest tube to remove excess air, allowing lung re-expansion.

PO—abbreviation from the Latin per os, meaning by mouth.

Positioning—intervention by a physical or occupational therapist to assist in muscular development of the infant. Includes the use of splints, braces, padding, or sandbagging to change and maintain a position of the body for an extended period of time.

Positive end—expiratory pressure (PEEP)-referent for a respirator providing consistent pressure to the lungs to prevent collapse during respiration.

PPD—see percussion and postural drainage.

Preeclampsia—the condition of high blood pressure, protein in the urine, and edema in pregnant women following 24 weeks of gestation that may necessitate early delivery to protect the health of the mother and fetus.

Premature—the birth of an infant prior to 37 weeks gestation.

Prenatal development—fetal growth and maturation that occurs in utero throughout gestation.

Prone—position in which the body is lying horizontal and face down.

Proprioceptive stimuli—elicitation of physical movement sensation and posture awareness, enabling body orientation to position in space without the aid of visual cues.

Proximo distal development—the neurological development of the infant that begins central to the body and moves outward.

Pseudmonas—a gram-negative bacteria often found in neonatal intensive care patients that may cause urinary tract infections as well as meningitis, may be resistant to antibiotic treatment, and requires contact isolation to prevent its spread.

Pulmonary hypertension—the abnormal condition of high pressure within the blood flow between the heart and lungs where blood is oxygenated and carbon dioxide removed.

Pulmonary insufficiency of the premature (PIP)—respiratory distress resulting from immature lungs and lack of surfactant, affecting primarily very young premature infants.

Pulmonary interstitial emphysema (PIE)—existence of bubbles of air pushed out of the alveoli between layers of lung tissue.

PVL—see periventricular leukomalacia.

Q (also q, qq)—an abbreviation for each or every.

qd (also qqd)—an abbreviation meaning every day.

qid (also qds)—an abbreviation meaning four times each day.

Rapid eye movement sleep (REM)—the state of sleep in which dreaming occurs, usually lasting a few minutes to half an hour, generally occurring at the beginning of an infant's sleep cycle, and detectable by electrodes placed on the skin surrounding the eye to record contractions of the eye muscles.

RDS—see respiratory distress syndrome.

Reciprocity—the two-way aspect of interaction in social communication.

Reflexive smile—involuntary movement in response to a stimulus without the consciousness of the infant. Observed from birth.

REM—see rapid eye movement sleep.

Respirator—a mechanical apparatus used to assist breathing.

Respiratory distress syndrome (RDS)—see hyaline membrane disease.

Respiratory syncytial virus (RSV)—a virus, sometimes fatal in infants, that can cause bronchiolitis, bronchopneumonia, and the common cold.

Resuscitate—the use of artificial respiration, cardiac massage, and correction of acid-base imbalance in order to restore cardiac and pulmonary function.

Retina—the soft, semitransparent, nervous tissue membrane of the eye that receives then transmits external images to the brain through the optic nerve.

Retinopathy of prematurity (ROP)—abnormal growth of blood vessels in the eye due to incomplete blood vessel development at the time of birth that must complete development outside of the protection of the womb.

Retracting—the process of shrinking, shortening, or pulling back.

Retrolental fibroplasia—the abnormal development of fibrous tissue behind the eye lens in neonates, caused by extensive administration of high-concentrations of oxygen, that leads to blindness.

Rhythm—the duration and patterns of beats and pulses.

Room air—the air naturally occurring in the environment, such as in the neonatal intensive care unit. It indicates that the infant is not receiving additional oxygen support but may be receiving room air via a nasal canula to aid breathing..

Rooting reflex—the normal response of newborns, usually fading by 3 to 4 months of age, to turn the head, when the facial cheek is stroked beside the mouth, in the direction of the stroking stimulus and begin sucking.

ROP—see retinopathy of prematurity.

RSV—see respiratory syncytial virus.

Scalp IV—an intravenous line placed in the infant's scalp where veins are more prominent and where it is less likely to be pulled out by the child.

Septic work-up—comprehensive evaluation of cultures (lab tests in which microorganisms and cells are cultivated) performed to determine the presence of infection caused by pyogenic (pus-producing) microorganisms.

Sensory perception—the awareness of auditory, visual, gustatory, olfactory, and tactile stimuli.

Shunt—a tube creating an artificial passage between two areas of the body to drain fluid.

SIDS—see sudden infant death syndrome.

Skin-to-skin contact—see kangaroo care.

SLD—see developmental disabilities associated with prematurity.

Small for gestational age (SGA)—neonate with length and weight less than the 10th percentile of infants appropriate for gestational age, regardless of pre-, full-, or post-term delivery.

Special education—instruction designed to meet the needs of exceptional students.

Specific learning disability—see developmental disabilities associated with prematurity.

Spina bifida—a congenital anomaly in which the bony spinal column fails to close completely during fetal development.

Spinal tap—see lumbar puncture.

Splints—a flexible or rigid device used to support or immobilize any body part in orthopedic treatment.

Startle reflex—see moro reflex.

Step reflex—the natural response in newborns, also called the dance reflex, that is usually replaced by more deliberate movement by 3 to 6 weeks of age, in which the infant approximates a walking movement when held in an erect position with feet touching a solid surface.

Strabismus—misalignment of the eyes resulting in their pointing in two different directions (e.g., cross-eyed).

Subarachnoid hemorrhage (SAH)—an intracranial hemorrhage that occurs in between the arachnoid and pia mater membranes on the brain's surface, extending into the brain when severe.

Suck reflex—an involuntary reflex which develops before 36 gestational weeks. An infant produces a strong sucking action when an object is placed in the mouth by extending the tongue over the lower gum, and raising the lower jaw.

Suck/swallow/breathe coordinated response—a sequence of well-coordinated responses that allow the infant to nipple or breast feed without choking.

Suctioning—the procedure of aspiration a fluid or gas by reduction of air pressure, generally produced mechanically.

Sudden infant death syndrome (SIDS)—the non-contagious, non-hereditary, sudden, and unexpected death of unknown cause of a healthy, typically developing infant during sleep that is the greatest cause of death of infants between the age of 2 weeks and 1 year, with incidence of 1 in every 300 to 350 births; prevention includes supine placement for sleep.

Supine—position in which the body is lying horizontally on the back.

Surfactant—the substance produced by the lungs that prevents the alveoli from collapsing and clinging together, a manufactured version (survanta) of which is administered to premature infants with immature lungs.

Swaddling—the technique of tightly wrapping a neonate to provide comfort.

Tachycardia—rapid heart rate.

Tachypnea—rapid respiration.

Term infant—infant born at full term between 38 and 42 weeks gestation.

Testosterone—an androgenic hormone produced in the adrenal cortex and ovaries and in larger amounts in the testes of the male.

TID (also tid, tdd)—an abbreviation meaning three times each day.

Total parenteral nutrition (TPN)—sugar, minerals, vitamins, and proteins resembling what would have been provided through the placenta and umbilical line that is provided to the premature infant intravenously.

TPN—see total parenteral nutrition.

Tracheostomy—surgical opening created in the windpipe that extends from the throat to the bronchial tubes, called the trachea, so that airflow can reach the lungs when an obstruction exists in the throat, the procedure for which is called tracheotomy.

Tracking ability—the skill used to visually follow objects as they move in, out, and within the field of vision or to focus attention across time on a moving sound source.

Trimester—one of the three period divisions of gestation, lasting approximately 3 months each.

UAC—see umbilical artery catheter.

Ultrasound—a procedure in which an image is obtained from high-frequency sound waves, used in fetal monitoring and internal organ assessment.

Umbilical artery catheter (UAC)—a thin tube inserted into the umbilical artery of the neonate used for emergency delivery of medication or fluids, for exchange blood transfusion, and to obtain blood samples.

Umbilical cord—the approximately 2 feet long and ½ inch diameter structure connecting the fetus to the placenta that supplies nutritional, immunological, hormonal, and blood supply needs to the developing fetus.

Umbilical venous catheter (UVC)—a thin tube inserted into an umbilical vein of the neonate used for delivery of medication or fluids and to obtain blood samples.

Upper respiratory infection (URI)—inflammation of the airways above the larynx caused by virus or bacteria.

URI—see upper respiratory infection.

Urinary tract infection (UTI)—inflammation of the kidneys, ureters, bladder, or urethra caused by bacteria and treated with antibiotics.

UTI—see urinary tract infection.

UVC—see umbilical venous catheter.

Vagus nerve—the 10th pair of cranial nerves that assist in control of heart rate and rhythms and digestion.

Vein catheter—any catheter placed in a vein (e.g., umbilical venous catheter).

Ventilator—device used to assist respiration and provide positive-pressure breathing.

Vital signs (VS)—body temperature, pulse, and respiratory rate.

VS—see vital signs.

Weaning—the process of gradually withdrawing the use of a ventilator on which the infant has become dependent.

Appendix

Metric Conversion Table
LENGTH: Inches to Centimeters

1 inch Increments
To obtain centimeters equivalent to 22 inches, read 20 on the top scale and 2 on the side scale which equals 55.9 cm

Inches	**0**	**10**	**20**	**30**	**40**
0	0	25.4	50.8	76.2	101.6
1	2.5	27.9	53.3	78.7	104.1
2	5.1	30.5	55.9	81.3	106.7
3	7.6	33.0	58.4	83.8	109.2
4	10.2	35.6	61.0	86.4	111.8
5	12.7	38.1	63.5	88.9	114.3
6	15.2	40.6	66.0	91.4	116.8
7	17.8	43.2	68.6	94.0	119.4
8	20.3	45.7	71.1	96.5	121.9
9	22.9	48.3	73.7	99.1	124.5

One-Quarter (1/4) inch Increments To obtain centimeters equivalent to 14 ¾ inches, read 14 on top scale and ¾ on side scale which equals 37.5 cm

Inches	**10**	**11**	**12**	**13**	**14**	**15**
0	25.4	27.9	30.5	33.0	35.6	38.1
¼	26.0	28.6	31.1	33.7	36.2	38.7
½	26.7	29.2	31.8	34.3	36.8	39.4
¾	27.3	29.8	32.4	34.9	37.5	40.0

Inches	**16**	**17**	**18**	**19**	**20**	**21**
0	40.6	43.2	45.7	48.3	50.8	53.3
¼	41.3	43.8	46.4	48.9	51.4	54.0
½	41.9	44.5	47.0	49.5	52.1	54.6
¾	42.5	45.1	47.6	50.2	52.7	55.2

Above table based on 1 inch=2.54 centimeters. Items rounded up one decimal when second decimal is 5 or greater.

Metric Conversion Table
WEIGHT: Pounds to Grams

OUNCES	POUNDS 0	1	2	3	4	5	6	7	8	9	10	11	12	13	14
0	0	454	907	1361	1814	2268	2722	3175	3629	4082	4536	4990	5443	5897	6350
1	28	482	936	1389	1843	2296	2750	3203	3657	4111	4564	5018	5471	5925	6379
2	57	510	964	1417	1871	2325	2778	3232	3685	4139	4593	5046	5500	5953	6407
3	85	539	992	1446	1899	2353	2807	3260	3714	4167	4621	5075	5528	5982	6435
4	113	567	1021	1474	1928	2381	2835	3289	3742	4196	4649	5103	5557	6010	6464
5	142	595	1049	1503	1956	2410	2863	3317	3770	4224	4678	5131	5585	6038	6492
6	170	624	1077	1531	1984	2438	2892	3345	3799	4252	4706	5160	5613	6067	6520
7	198	652	1106	1559	2013	2466	2920	3374	3827	4281	4734	5188	5642	6095	6549
8	227	680	1134	1588	2041	2495	2948	3402	3856	4309	4763	5216	5670	6123	6577
9	255	709	1162	1616	2070	2523	2977	3430	3884	4337	4791	5245	5698	6152	6605
10	283	737	1191	1644	2098	2551	3005	3459	3912	4366	4819	5273	5727	6180	6634
11	312	765	1219	1673	2126	2580	3033	3487	3941	4394	4848	5301	5755	6209	6662
12	340	794	1247	1701	2155	2608	3062	3515	3969	4423	4876	5330	5783	6237	6690
13	369	822	1276	1729	2183	2637	3090	3544	3997	4451	4904	5358	5812	6265	6719
14	397	850	1304	1758	2211	2665	3118	3572	4026	4478	4933	5386	5840	6294	6747
15	425	879	1332	1786	2240	2693	3147	3600	4054	4508	4961	5415	5868	6322	6776

Note: 1 pound (lb) = 453.59237 grams (g); 1 ounce (oz) = 28.349523 grams; 1000 grams = 1kilogram (k). Gram equivalents have been rounded to whole numbers by adding one when the first decimal place is 5 or greater.

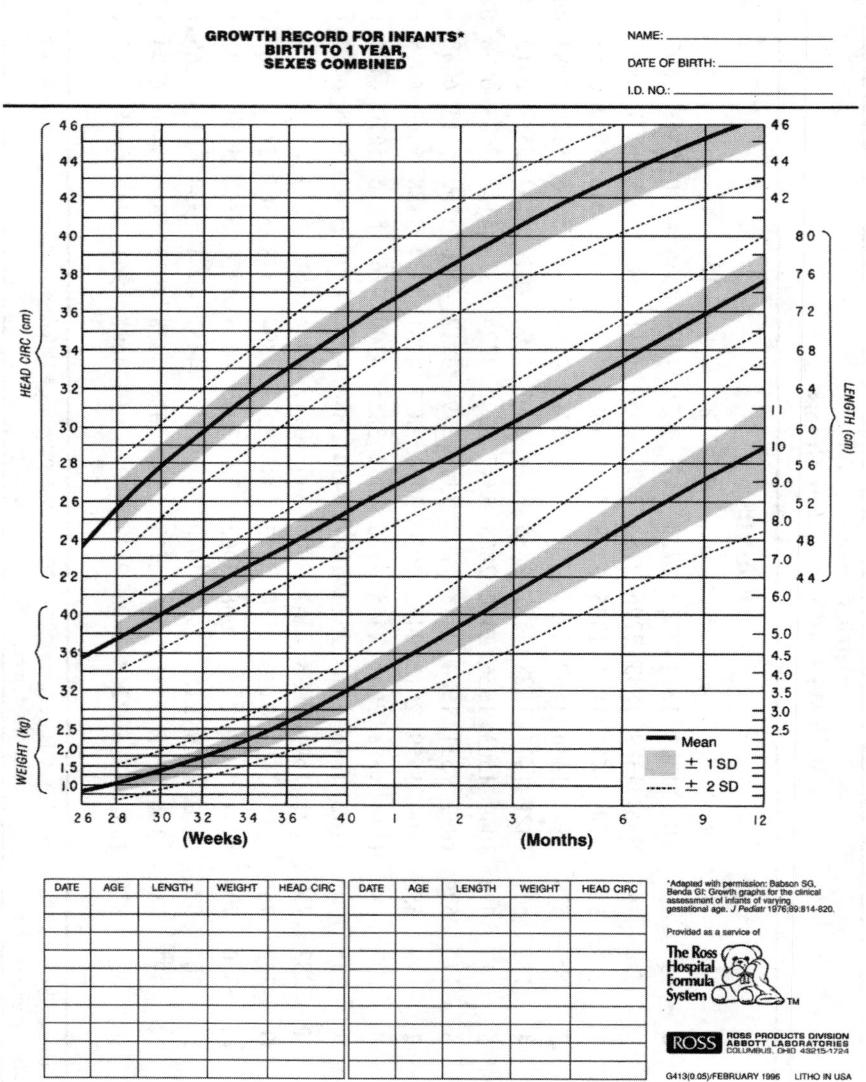

DATE	AGE	LENGTH	WEIGHT	HEAD CIRC	DATE	AGE	LENGTH	WEIGHT	HEAD CIRC

MATURATIONAL ASSESSMENT OF GESTATIONAL AGE (New Ballard Score)

NAME ____________________ SEX ____________________

HOSPITAL NO. ____________________ BIRTH WEIGHT ____________________

RACE ____________________ LENGTH ____________________

DATE/TIME OF BIRTH ____________________ HEAD CIRC. ____________________

DATE/TIME OF EXAM ____________________ EXAMINER ____________________

AGE WHEN EXAMINED ____________________

APGAR SCORE: 1 MINUTE __________ 5 MINUTES __________ 10 MINUTES __________

NEUROMUSCULAR MATURITY

NEUROMUSCULAR MATURITY SIGN	SCORE							RECORD SCORE HERE
	-1	0	1	2	3	4	5	
POSTURE								
SQUARE WINDOW (Wrist)	>90°	90°	60°	45°	30°	0°		
ARM RECOIL		180°	140°-180°	110°-140°	90°-110°	<90°		
POPLITEAL ANGLE	180°	160°	140°	120°	100°	90°	<90°	
SCARF SIGN								
HEEL TO EAR								
							TOTAL NEUROMUSCULAR MATURITY SCORE	

SCORE

Neuromuscular __________

Physical __________

Total __________

MATURITY RATING

score	weeks
-10	20
-5	22
0	24
5	26
10	28
15	30
20	32
25	34
30	36
35	38
40	40
45	42
50	44

PHYSICAL MATURITY

PHYSICAL MATURITY SIGN	SCORE							RECORD SCORE HERE
	-1	0	1	2	3	4	5	
SKIN	sticky friable transparent	gelatinous red translucent	smooth pink visible veins	superficial peeling &/or rash, few veins	cracking pale areas rare veins	parchment deep cracking no vessels	leathery cracked wrinkled	
LANUGO	none	sparse	abundant	thinning	bald areas	mostly bald		
PLANTAR SURFACE	heel-toe 40-50 mm:-1 <40 mm:-2	>50 mm no crease	faint red marks	anterior transverse crease only	creases ant. 2/3	creases over entire sole		
BREAST	imperceptible	barely perceptible	flat areola no bud	stippled areola 1-2 mm bud	raised areola 3-4 mm bud	full areola 5-10 mm bud		
EYE/EAR	lids fused loosely: -1 tightly: -2	lids open pinna flat stays folded	sl. curved pinna; soft; slow recoil	well-curved pinna; soft but ready recoil	formed & firm instant recoil	thick cartilage ear stiff		
GENITALS (Male)	scrotum flat, smooth	scrotum empty faint rugae	testes in upper canal rare rugae	testes descending few rugae	testes down good rugae	testes pendulous deep rugae		
GENITALS (Female)	clitoris prominent & labia flat	prominent clitoris & small labia minora	prominent clitoris & enlarging minora	majora & minora equally prominent	majora large minora small	majora cover clitoris & minora		
							TOTAL PHYSICAL MATURITY SCORE	

GESTATIONAL AGE (weeks)

By dates __________

By ultrasound __________

By exam __________

Reference
Ballard JL, Khoury JC, Wedig K, et al: New Ballard Score, expanded to include extremely premature infants. *J Pediatr* 1991; 119:417-423. Reprinted by permission of Dr Ballard and Mosby-Year Book, Inc.

Index of Names and Subjects

B

C

D

E

F

G

K

L

M

N

O

P

R

S

T

U

V

W

Y

Z

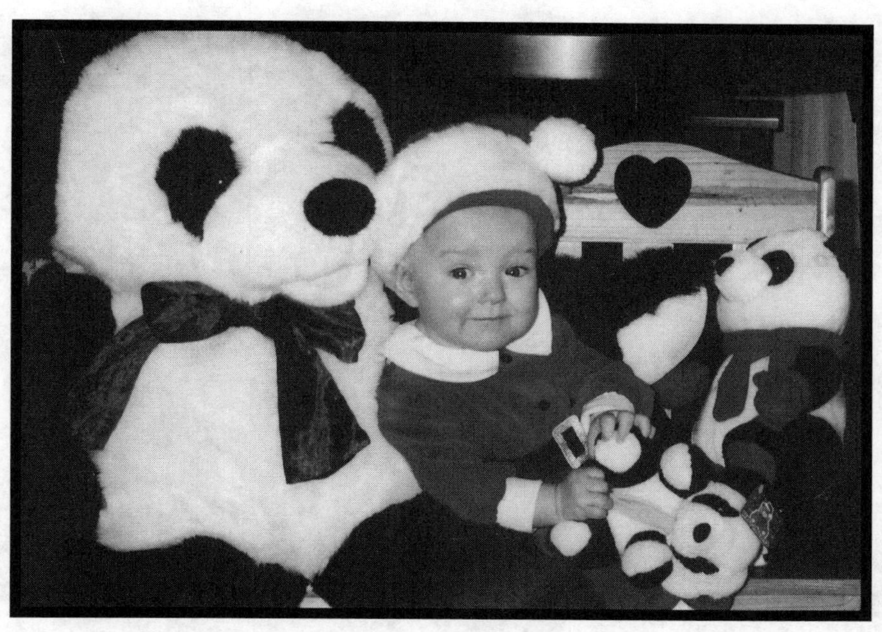

Adorable Libby enjoying her first Christmas and almost ready for her first birthday, though she will be only 9 months adjusted gestational age at that time.